COFFEE ON SUNDAYS

By Barbara Lawson Reesor O.T. Reg., CM

Cover is original artwork by the author Barbara Lawson Reesor.

"Coffee on Sundays," by Barbara Lawson Reesor. ISBN 978-1-60264-169-3.

Published 2008 by Virtualbookworm.com Publishing Inc., P.O. Box 9949, College Station, TX 77842, US.

Manufactured in the United States of America.

Table of Contents

Dedication

This book is dedicated to Dr. Myra Rodrigues. I will be forever grateful to her for her role in the creation, support of and completion of this book.

Introduction

This is the true story of "Erica Chase, a.k.a. Rikki", who was confined against her will to an institution for the "retarded", an unpleasant term used at the time, for her entire adolescent years, during the 1970's and 1980's. This was not because she had misbehaved or broken the law, but because she was blind and disabled and her parents were unable to care for her.

The tragic thing about this, first and foremost, was that Rikki was not mentally disabled and second, that there were many more like her in the institution.

This story begins at a Rehabilitation Centre in Ontario, Canada, where Rikki was the first resident to be sent for a short evaluation to determine her potential for treatment. This was in accordance with a new government policy to try to reduce the huge population in these institutions. It was at Rehab where it was discovered that Rikki was not mentally disabled. Nevertheless, she was sent back to the institution because, due to her double disability of blindness and cerebral palsy, she did not fit existing criteria for placement anywhere else.

Following Rikki's return to the institution, the story introduces a number of other residents like her who were selected for a special ward for blind residents. Through them, readers experience the anger, frustration, despair and apathy of many of these young people. Readers also vicariously celebrate when many of the residents discover themselves and a life of opportunity outside the institution. While characters names have been changed to protect individuals, the situations described were pervasive in Government institutions in the late 1970s and early 1980s and actually did happen.

This book supports the Ontario government's intention to phase out these institutions in favor of community-based group homes. The story sheds some light on the controversy inherent in all large institutions. Furthermore, it shows how blindness coupled with other disabilities can lead to a mistaken diagnosis, and how confinement over a long period without education or an activity program can disguise true ability. Finally, it is a story about one aspect of Occupational Therapy, the only medical profession that concentrates more on the ability of the patient than the disability.

This story depicts the author's role in releasing Rikki from the institution and into suitable Rehabilitation Services. She went on to help others as the Founder and President of the Therapeutic and Educational Living Centres for the Blind, which were named TELCI House and REESOR House. TELCI was the first Cheshire home for the blind in North America. In 1984, she was awarded the Order of Canada in recognition of her work with blind, multi-handicapped adults.

PART 1 – THE REHAB CENTRE

Chapter 1

THE NEW PATIENT

"At one time there was practically no effective program in the field of mental retardation. Wherever possible the children were committed to institutions".
President John F. Kennedy
News Conference 17
October 11, 1961

The time has come to write down what happened, not that I will forget, because the events are still engraved as clearly on my mind as when they happened, but because it sometimes takes a while for things to fall into their true perspective. It takes time for the patterns to come into focus, and for all the non-essentials that might have seemed important at the time to fade into the background where they belong.

It was one of the hottest days in late July, 1970. I was a staff occupational therapist (O.T.) at the Rehabilitation Centre and was looking through a list of new admissions. My case load had recently been reduced as a result of several discharges, and therapists were expected to pick up new patients as soon as they were able to take them. It was five years since I had graduated from the university and completed my internship as an O.T. I liked the challenge of physical medicine.

Most of the patients in this fifty-bed active treatment centre were older people recovering from stroke, young men and women with spinal cord injuries from motor vehicle or sports accidents, a few with multiple sclerosis and other neurological problems. There were a few head injuries, some amputees and a number with arthritis. But while each patient had his own unique problems, the list of disabilities was usually predictable.

For this reason I was surprised when, looking over the list of new referrals in the secretary's office my eye fell on one that was different -- Erika Chase, age 19, diagnosis: total congenital blindness, cerebral palsy and mental retardation -- to have a three-week assessment only. I had often wondered why we had never had a blind patient at Rehab; surely blind people had health problems. I hung the clip-board back on its hook, nodded to the secretary on duty and slowly walked back past the treatment rooms to the occupational therapy office. What a devastating combination of disabilities. What would be the primary disability? Where would one start?

When I first came to Rehab, a year earlier, we had no full time physician. Several doctors came in once or twice a week, or as needed, to examine prospective patients for suitability for treatment. The patient was admitted or came in as an out- patient, and would be referred by the physician to various departments according to his or her needs, such as social work, psychology, speech pathology, physiotherapy, occupational therapy or nursing.

Dr. Pentland was our first resident physician. He had come in two weeks ago like a new broom. Popularity with the staff was not one of his priorities. He made it understood from the first day that he would not tolerate incompetence, and gave the impression that we were all incompetent until proved otherwise. Our Head O.T., Doreen Mason, was a capable medical administrator, and won her colours immediately with Dr Pentland.

Even at this time, in the early 1970's, Rehabilitation Medicine was a new field and had not been fully accepted or appreciated by the medical profession. It was, in fact, described by some physicians as the lowest rung on the medical ladder. Even the title, "physiatrist", meaning "specialist in physical medicine", was frequently confused with "psychiatrist". For that matter, occupational therapy was usually confused with physiotherapy, (now called physical therapy), or it was assumed that it was merely a hospital-based form of recreation and handicrafts.

The O.T. office door was ajar, meaning that Doreen was still there, although it was almost five o'clock. I knocked and walked in. She was sitting at her desk writing a report, papers and files in neat stacks in front of her. Doreen was the epitome of the career therapist, crisp white blouse with red O.T. crest, dark green skirt and cardigan, and brown shoes with sensible heels. The O.T. uniform had evolved from the original green military style with the starched collar and Sam Brown belt, but had retained the green skirt colour and the same crest.

"I'd like to pick up that blind patient, Doreen, if it's O.K," I said. "It's only a three week assessment and it should be fairly straight-forward. I don't suppose the patient has any potential, but it looks interesting, for a change. What an incredible diagnosis -- C.P., blindness and mental retardation."

"It's all right with me, Sally," said Doreen. "But try to see her right away. Dr. Pentland wants a fairly quick assessment. She's the first patient from that huge centre for the retarded out at Burnside. Do you remember when I went out with a team to assess the needs there? They're trying to reduce their population. For this reason, though, it's essential that we understand that she's to go right back after the assessment. There's no placement problem. What's your case load like?"

"It was heavy last week, but I'm down to twelve now, and some come for treatment only two or three days a week. I'd like to take her."

"O.K., but be ready to present your initial report at next week's conference, won't you?"

"No problem, Doreen," I said. "See you tomorrow."

Even the night offered little relief from the hot spell and the next day dawned hot and clear again. The Rehab building was old, with no air conditioning, and while the dark corridors gave the illusion of coolness in contrast to the brightness outside, they were close and airless. Nevertheless, Gerry, the elevator operator, looked fresh in his pale blue uniform jacket.

"Another warm day today, Miss," he said as he closed the doors. "When's it going to end?"

"I guess we need a big storm, Gerry. Take me up to four please."

It was cooler on the fourth floor. The four beds on the ward were empty, neatly made, each with its own bedside table and chair. The only sound was the large floor fan rippling the curtains in the summer heat. Sitting quietly alone in the far left hand corner of the room, Erika Chase seemed to be stuffed into her too-small wheelchair. She was hunched forward, head on chest, arms in lap, knees over-bent, so that she gave the impression of being perfectly round. How very round she looked, not child-like or old, but somehow ageless and sexless.

"Hello," I said, "I'm Miss Wallace, your Occupational Therapist. You must be Erika Chase."

I was standing on her right side. Suddenly her head shot up and her face turned away from me, towards the window, her left arm groping around for me on the wrong side. "I'm over here," I said, taking her hand.

"Yes Madam, that's me," she replied. "My name's Erika, but everyone calls me Rikki, spelled with two Ks. I just came in last night." Her voice was strident and too loud, as though she thought I was ten feet away.

I was surprised by the clarity of her voice. It was almost boy-like, and the articulation appeared to be unaffected by the cerebral palsy. This could only mean that the C.P was not as severe as it appeared, yet I would have expected a cerebral palsy patient with this degree of physical disability to have a severe speech problem.

"I know," I replied. "I'm pleased to meet you. I'll be working with you every day. I'm one of a team of four or five other therapists, and we'll all be asking you a lot of questions. Do you know what an O.T. is?"

"Yes Madam. The doctor told me. And I want to tell you something. I will do whatever you want -- no matter what. Do you understand what I mean? Let's get started. You just give the orders. But, what's your first name? I always go by first names. It's friendlier, don't you think? I'm blind, you know, but don't let that bother you. I see my way and you see yours. We're going to get along fine. You just give the orders and I'll do the work. Nothing's too hard for me."

I told her my name was Sally. What's the harm? Informality might be better with this patient.

"O.K. Sally," she replied. "Let's get goin'."

"It's going to be another hot day to-day Rikki. Do you mind the heat?"

"Madam… I mean, Sally, I love it. The reason is because I love everything about this place. I'm so happy to be here I could cry. I probably will cry a lot. I always do when I'm happy. I like to sing too. Do you like to sing?"

"Well, I like singing, but I haven't much of a singing voice."

"I have. I sing all the time. What would you like to hear?"

"First I have to do an assessment, Rikki. Do you know what an assessment is?"

"It means you ask me to do a lot of things. I'll try, but if I fail will they send me back?"

"No Rikki. It's not like that at all. It's not something you pass or fail. It's just a way for us to find out what you can do. Now there's something I want to tell you, Rikki. You're blind, and you're my first blind patient, so I can't pretend to know much about blindness. If I'm going to help you, you'll have to help me in return."

"It's a deal. And Madam… Sally… *you listen to me.* I'm blind, but I've always been blind, so I don't mind it. If you gave me two eyes right now I wouldn't know what to do with them. Sort of like getting a third leg. Do you understand? So let's get on with it."

What a lot of insight this girl had. Within the first five minutes she was telling me not to waste pity on her and I was beginning to be aware of something that was to become more evident to me as we progressed -- that Rikki's appearance was misleading. If I shut my eyes and just talked to her I got a different impression, because she looked so disabled. Her facial expression and gestures, as well as her overall appearance, were unattractive and unacceptable by normal standards. Yet, in spite of the raucous voice, something else was coming through. Her gestures were irritatingly inappropriate. Her hair, greasy and uncombed, covered her eyes. Her complexion was sallow. Her figure was shapeless, except for that curious roundness. But there was also something appealing about her.

I had the strangest feeling of incongruity. In less than five minutes Rikki had put me at ease and initiated the action. She was almost reversing the roles. I had expected an impossible case, someone who was totally dependent, mentally and physically, and probably uneducable and helpless. Instead, I had found someone who was well motivated, not a bit shy, cooperative, and who demonstrated keen insight into her blindness.

I wrote a note on my clipboard -- Assets: clear voice, much like a boy's, no articulation problem, motivation high, not shy, incessant talker but limited vocabulary, repetitive. Rikki was repeating over and over how happy she was to be here.

"Tell me something about yourself Rikki," I said. "How old are you?"

"I'm nineteen," she said. "My parents had to put me away when I was eight because my mum got sick and my dad was away a lot and I was getting too heavy to lift. They told me I was going away to school, but when I got there I found that I was in this place with the retarded. Well ..." she took a deep breath... "It's hard to tell you what that was like… sort of lonely, you know. There was no one really who could talk to me, except the staff, and they were always too busy. The residents talked, but it wasn't words, just yellin' and hollerin', yellin' and hollerin' away, without any meaning. I like the quiet here, and now I can have my radio all the time. I never could there. It always had to be locked up because the others would break it."

"Did your family go to see you often?"

"Oh yes, sometimes on long week-ends. And we had Parents' Day once a year when they would come. But my mum hated coming. It always made her cry. I wish I could stay here and never go back there."

"Rikki, you know this is just an assessment, don't you? You'll be here for only three weeks. Then you'll go back. That's the arrangement."

"Well.... I'm just not going to think about it. I'm going to enjoy myself for three whole weeks and work like the blazes. I'm a real worker, you'll see."

"OK show me what you can do. Can you stand up?"

"Well… no… not stand. I never have. My knees are bent and won't go straight. Do you want me to try? Maybe if you help ---"

"No, not now, not until we get you a better wheelchair and a transfer belt to put around your waist so you won't fall. Is this your own wheelchair?"

"Not really. It's just one they lent me. My dad asked them to get me one three years ago, but every time a new one came in it went to someone else. I guess they don't think you need one when you're blind.

"We'll lend you one while you're here, Rikki. You're going to need a wheelchair with removable arms and good brakes. This is a child's chair and it's too tippy and small for you now. Can you dress yourself at all?"

"Someone always dresses me, but I'd like to learn if you'd teach me."

"What about eating?" I asked. "Can you use a knife and fork?"

"I can use a spoon, but I usually use my fingers because I don't know what I'm eating if I can't feel it, and it just slides off the plate. How could I use a knife and fork?"

"Can you reach your feet Rikki?"

"Oh my, no. When I'm on the bed my feet are quite far away. If I could hear them I would know about where they are. But I'm not very good at pushing up on the bed either, because I'm afraid of falling out. I might be able to reach my feet sitting in the wheelchair, but it's tippy, and I haven't got a seat belt, so I'd probably fall right out of the chair."

"You're right about that. Can you sit up by yourself if you grab the pipes?"

"Well, you see, I've only got the use of my left hand, so I might pull too hard and fall off the bed. I've never been allowed to try. Maybe you could show me how I could do it."

Rikki was well oriented as to time and place. She knew what day it was, approximately what time it was and why she was here. She did not know how to tell the time with a Braille clock. She could spell her name and she could count to ten by rote. Apart from that, her assessment scores on the chart were all zeroes. I wrote in summary: *An almost totally dependent nineteen year old girl, highly motivated and articulate, congenitally blind, spastic right arm and both legs, speech not affected by the cerebral palsy but rather juvenile, repetitive, well oriented - needs wheelchair.*

I said good-bye again as I was leaving so that Rikki could hear me going out the door. I was afraid she would never stop talking. What a strange case, quite different from what I'd expected. At face value, or on paper, this girl had all the odds against her, but somehow something was contradicting the facts of total helplessness. She did not behave like an invalid. She had hope, determination, courage and candor in larger quantities than many so-called "normal" patients.

As I read Rikki's chart in the ward office I became more and more convinced that what I was reading was different from what I saw. Could it be possible that someone had made a mistake? Medical people often admit that they sometimes have "gut feelings" about a case, a kind of intuition that often proves to be valuable in diagnosis and treatment, and I had a hunch that this was going to be no ordinary case. Little did I know that those next few weeks were going to change my life.

Chapter 2

IN THE BALANCE

"Confinement and anxiety will subdue the stoutest hearts."
Charles Dickens

I was not ready for the case conference on Friday. In only one week Rikki's admission had generated controversy among the entire staff. While this was only an initial conference, it was important because it would set forth the strengths and weaknesses of the patient to determine prognosis and, in Rikki's case, I felt that this was premature. At the same time the conference gave an opportunity for members of the treatment team to compare findings, and Rikki would, by now, have been seen by all members of the team; physician, nurse, physiotherapist, occupational therapist, speech pathologist, social worker and psychologist.

I still had an hour before the conference, so I went to the cafeteria for a cup of coffee. Winding my way through the crowded tables, I found a vacant seat beside George McWhittie, one of the psychologists. At once he started to talk about Rikki.

"She shouldn't be here," he said. "This isn't a place for the retarded. We have a waiting list as long as your arm and we should be taking people who can benefit. Working with the retarded is a dead-end street."

"Have you ever worked with the retarded, George?" I asked.

"Only a short time," he replied, "when I was a student. But I couldn't get much interested because I kept thinking what difference does it make what level they're functioning on if they're retarded anyway?"

"It's easier for the staff, for one thing," I said, "if they can become independent in self-care."

"Nonsense," he replied. "It's harder for the staff. It takes longer for them to dress and wash themselves. In fact the staff tries to prevent them from learning too much, because then they might start to think about doing other things for themselves, and that makes it much harder. That's when you get all the behavior problems. Besides, everyone knows that brain damage goes along with Cerebral Palsy (C.P.). C.P. is a condition, not an illness that can be treated. It doesn't change. It's just a waste of time and money to try to train a C.P."

"But George," I protested, "I know many C.P.s who have above normal intelligence. I even know of one who became a physician. How can you make a statement like that?"

"Be sensible, Sally," he replied. "That girl is not only retarded, but she has C.P. and she's spent her whole life with the retarded. We know that a normal child can actually *become* retarded if left with them for many years. She's nineteen. It's too late to do anything now. She's too old to learn, so you might as well face it. Rehab centers are for people who can benefit from rehabilitation, and I can tell you, even before we test that girl, that it's a waste of time. But we can't do it at least till next week, so the rest of you will have plenty of time to get your reports done."

After coffee I went back to the ward where Carol, a physiotherapist, was discussing Rikki's case with one of the nurses. "She should have been able to walk," Carol was saying. "The C.P. is actually quite mild, but it's exaggerated because of the blindness, and she's had no treatment or exercise for so many years that I doubt if we'll be able to stretch those hamstrings enough for her to stand up. It's a real shame."

"Well," said the nurse, "It's easy to feel sorry for the poor kid, but pity won't help her. Here comes the O.T. Sally, I wish you'd hurry and teach Rikki to sit on the toilet. She's always been taught to use a bedpan, like an invalid. How independent do you think she can be?"

"She has no idea of positioning yet," I replied. "She can't even sit alone on the side of the bed, so be careful when you move her. But don't lift her. It's unnecessary. I know you're working on the same thing Carol. I'm going to use a Velcro-fastened transfer belt to move her from one surface to the other until she gets the idea. I think we can teach her to transfer if we tell her what to do step by step. She's already learned to roll over and she can almost sit up alone. Every day we're doing exercises on the bed to increase strength and balance. What are you finding in physio, Carol?"

"We haven't finished assessing yet," said Carol. "We'll wait till after the conference this morning before starting any actual treatment in case she doesn't stay. Do you notice that she has a peculiar odor? Do all retarded people smell? It makes me sick. I hope they discharge her. That old wheelchair she came in is positively antique, and dangerous too. She could tip right over backwards in it. I hope you can spare one from O.T. to lend her."

"Yes, but I'm going to assess her for a new chair. She certainly shouldn't go back in that old thing."

"But Sally, you'll never get it in time. It takes three months or more. The last one we ordered took closer to six months because you've got to arrange the funding. But I guess you know what you're doing. See you at the case conference in about ten minutes."

The conference did not go well. I found myself on the defensive. What was this hostility against this girl? I had never experienced this before at Rehab

Dr. Pentland was speaking: "We are a community service. We have been asked to assess this severely handicapped girl over a period of three weeks. At the end of that time we will *endeavour* to instruct the staff at the institution in how to manage her. They have asked for help, but they are not receptive to rehabilitation. The institution is designed to provide custodial care for the mentally retarded, yet they seem to have a considerable number of physically disabled residents. Their staff is static, there is practically no turn-over. Many of the staff have been there for years, and are not ready to change their ideas. You may now present your initial assessment reports."

Physiotherapy usually led off. The report gave a guarded prognosis, describing severe limitation of movement in the right arm and lower extremities. The therapist felt that the decision as to whether or not the patient would be able to walk was premature until icing and stretching had been tried.

The speech therapist reported that there was no pathological problem in receptive and expressive language or articulation, but the nasal quality and lack of modulation in the voice, as well as verbal repetition and limited vocabulary were probably due to institutionalization. The patient did not require speech therapy.

The social worker confirmed that plans to return the patient to the institution presented no problems, because this had been arranged before admission. The psychology report was not available.

My report generated the most discussion. "We must have a suitable wheelchair for this patient, in order to test her transfer potential. She has never been taught to transfer and I think I can teach her."

"You're not being paid to conjecture," stated Dr Pentland. "What makes you think you can obtain a new wheelchair for this patient within the next week, when everyone else takes three to six months?"

"I feel that this delay is unnecessary," I replied. "The whole future of this patient may depend on getting that chair. I'm only asking for permission to try."

"Do you have anything else to report?"

"Yes," I said. "I don't think this patient is retarded."

"That is not your department. What about her self-care. Get on with your report! You are wasting the time of this conference."

I felt intimidated by a doctor for the first time in my career, although it was Dr. Pentland's nature to be provocative with therapists. But it made me angry. I found myself on the defensive and decided to present as much of my report as he would permit.

"I can't test this girl by existing standards," I said. "She doesn't fit the report forms. I think that many of the skills she lacks she could learn. I'll need more time. I'm asking for three weeks extension of assessment time and permission to order a wheelchair."

Dr. Pentland thumbed through the pages of the chart again. "The occupational therapist has raised the question of psychological functioning which cannot be discussed because we have no report. I want a complete neuro-psychology report on this patient. Dr. Brough, do you see your way clear to providing such a report within a reasonable time?"

"Not before two weeks, at the earliest, maybe three," replied Dr. Brough. "I'll look into it right away."

"Very well Miss Wallace, you will have three weeks from today, and that wheelchair is to be ordered only on condition that it arrives in time to be useful. Next patient?"

I found refuge in Doreen's office. "What do you know about mental retardation, Doreen," I asked. "How do you decide if a person is retarded or not?"

"There are many types of retardation Sally," said Doreen. "Usually when a child fails to reach a certain developmental level at certain accepted ages and stages he's considered to be retarded, or developmentally delayed, as they call it now. His learning ability may stop at any age. For example, he may be thirty years old with a mental age of three."

"But what if a child is deprived of the opportunity to learn certain skills, like being in a wheelchair in an institution for the retarded for years, wouldn't that affect his developmental level? And if he were blind too?"

"I should think it would affect it a great deal. Have you contacted the Institute for the Blind? You should do that right away. I'll ask for a search of the literature for you. But don't get too carried away with this case." Doreen continued. "I should warn you, it's a kind of political thing, and we can't afford to get too involved with the institution."

I went to my desk and looked up the telephone number for Everest and Jennings in Middleton. This was the Head Office for the largest wheelchair company. I knew that I would have to by-pass the local agent to get a wheelchair in time. I spoke to the Manager who put me through to one of the dealers and explained the problem.

"Six months to get a chair? You've got to be kidding. Of course I can get you some action. I'll do better than that… I'll get you a chair. Is tomorrow O.K.? You bet your sweet life I will. I'll snatch it off the production line myself, and I'll even escort it personally to your Centre. Maybe you have a few more orders you'd like to fill. You've got the right man this time."

He was a typical salesman but he sounded capable and enthusiastic. He took down all the particulars; "Active Duty Lightweight sixteen inch seat, swing-aways, desk arms, any colour. That will run you about $500.00 with hospital discount. Who shall I bill it to?"

I knew if I waited for funding through social services there would be delays, so I found myself saying "bill it to me." I knew that funding would be found eventually through March of Dimes if no other way, or a service club would help out, but this search for funding often caused much of the long delay in providing patients with wheelchairs. Now I was really committed to teaching Rikki to transfer and time was limited. I wondered what had caused the blindness. Retrolental Fibroplasia -- what did that mean? No one seemed to know anything about it, not even the doctors. Could it be corrected? Would it respond to surgery, or transplant?

Suddenly it occurred to me that there were no eye reports on Rikki's file. I wondered why. Was it possible that she had never been seen by an eye specialist? What if something could be done to restore her vision? Why hadn't anyone mentioned this at the conference? I began to visualize the hospital room, Rikki with bandages being removed. What would her reaction be when she could see for the first time?

As a professional I had trained myself over the years not to carry my work home - never to mix business with pleasure. Professionals always had to be careful not to get emotionally involved with their patients, but I found myself thinking about Rikki on my way home, and I was looking forward more than ever to the next day.

Chapter 3

CROSSROADS

"Better one hour of a free life than forty years of slavery and imprisonment."
Rigas Feraios

For centuries the Aesculapian symbol of the serpent and the rod has represented the healing arts. Just as Aesculapius, (the world's first physician according to Greek mythology), was reputed to have the power to bring the dead to life, so medical ethics throughout history have proclaimed the philosophy of life and healing.

Euthanasia has never gained a foothold in western society, but it is only in recent years that the *quality* of life has been questioned, and the rights of an individual to live as normally and fully as possible have been defined, in Canada, in a human rights code. While the medical profession agrees that it is unethical as well as illegal to withdraw life support systems from severely handicapped babies, as Rikki was, it did not feel it was unethical to condemn her to a life as a "vegetable" in an institution far removed from the mainstream of society. Parents were assured that it would be better for the rest of the family, that she would not know the difference, and that she would be with "her own kind" and with staff who knew how best to look after her. Parents were invariably assured that permanent brain damage rendered the child helpless and "uneducable", without any follow-up to ascertain if in fact this was true.

A difficult situation then faces a therapist who becomes aware that the patient is capable of attaining more independence than the present environment will permit. Suspecting that the facilities the patient needs are not present in the community, should a therapist persist in training that individual, thereby creating a demand for services he cannot have, and raising his hopes and expectations?

I was having lunch with some of the staff in the dining room. The hum of fans and the buzz of conversation mingled with the clatter of dishes so that everyone had to strain to hear, but lunch time gave an opportunity to meet and talk shop.

Bev, an occupational therapist sitting opposite me, lit a cigarette and blew a puff of smoke across the table. I wished people would not smoke in the dining room, but non-smokers were outnumbered and it was never discussed.

"It's not my problem that there's no place for her to go in the community," I was saying. "And it's not her fault either."

"But Sally," replied Bev, "It's like training someone for a social level she can't fit into. You always have to keep in mind where she's going when she leaves."

"It's not the same thing at all, Bev," I said, "You don't think that way with a paraplegic who has to change his line of work and can't get into his house or his bathroom, but you're willing to tell Rikki that she mustn't try too hard because she'll have no place to live. It's like saying there's no point in doing emergency surgery on someone because he can't climb the stairs in his house after the surgery. If a paraplegic can't return to his home or his old job, don't we do everything we can to adapt his house and teach him to compensate in other ways?"

I turned to the person on my left, "Grace, you're a social worker. You know perfectly well that we do this for other patients. What's the difference with Rikki?"

"We have a placement problem for our quadriplegics too, Sally. You know that. And we have tried to find something for Rikki, but we can't find anything suitable. Her family can't take her, she's over age to be adopted or put in a foster home, the Agency residence for the Blind is not accessible and anyway, it's restricted to seniors, and Rikki can't manage alone in an apartment. What can we do except send her back to the institution? She can't stay here indefinitely. The conditions on admission were that she was to go back to the institution."

"Wouldn't it be better to send her to one of the nursing homes?" Asked Bev.

"They've refused her too," said Grace. "They all say their staff are not trained to take someone who is blind as well as wheelchair dependent."

Mildred, a speech therapist, who had been silent up to this point, now joined in the discussion, "If you want my opinion, Sally, you're playing with fire. You're raising the girl's expectations beyond what she can have, as well as making her dissatisfied with the institution, so she'll be more unhappy than ever when she goes back."

"She was unhappy when she came, Mildred. That's not my fault. She says she's treated as though she has no mind. She has no control over her environment at all. She can't make any decisions, has no money of her own, no possessions, hasn't even any real friends. She's desperately lonely. She's the only blind person on a ward with sighted retarded people who don't understand her blindness and can't communicate with her. No one has ever even read to her. Can you imagine what that must be like? It's unbelievable - in fact it's cruel. I'll be very surprised if that girl is actually retarded. Have you any idea how much she's learned already?"

"There's no doubt she's progressed a long way, Sally," said Bev. "But there's another problem you may not have thought of. She's getting very dependent on you. She talks about you on the ward all the time. Are you aware that she's practically driving the nurses nuts by saying, Sally says I don't have to do this, or that."

I was surprised. "No, I didn't know that. But if she's being manipulative, that's just another sign of her intelligence."

"Well, good luck to you Sally," said Bev. "I can see that you're getting very involved in this case and, after all, you are the prime therapist for Rikki and I am afraid we haven't been much help. Are you getting any help from the Agency for the Blind?"

"Not so far." I replied. "It's very strange. They seem to be putting us off. They've had her name on their registry since she was born, but they've never been near her. I've been trying to get one of those "talking book" machines I've heard about, but they're evasive about that too. I spoke to the District Administrator, but all he said was that there's a big run on them - no promises. I even arranged to meet with him a few days ago after work, but when I arrived he'd gone home and had forgotten about it."

"What about the library," asked Bev. "There are some ophthalmology journals there. There must be some American publications that might help."

"Yes, I've looked, and Doreen's done a search at two universities with medical school libraries. So far all we've been able to find concerns the single disability of blindness, or C.P., but there's nothing useful on a combined disability."

"Do you ever wish you'd never had this case?" Laughed Bev. "Sorry we can't be more help."

We picked up our trays, stacked them on the wagon and left the room. I had twenty minutes before I had to be on duty again so I went back to the library. This time I found a book about blind babies. Rikki wasn't a baby, but I thumbed through it just in case there might be something useful, and came across the following passages:

"Blind babies reach the normal stages of development more slowly than sighted babies... Parents of blind babies often feel alienated from friends and relatives who unwittingly make cruel remarks about the child." And then: "Blind babies receive information about their environment differently from sighted babies."

I began to read more carefully. "The blind should not be tested against norms designed for the sighted. Blindness can mask intelligence."

"Initially the blind infant has no control over the presence or absence of sound in his environment."

"Voices come out of nothingness and return to nothingness when they cease."

"The developmental process will be slower for the blind child because of lack of the visual half of distance perceptors."

"He is deprived of the stimulus of non-verbal language...."

"He is punished when he explores... Fear and danger delay his development."

"He may experience severe social rejection... *Such children may be misunderstood and are often mislabeled as mentally retarded.* Pressure from physician, friends and family often results in the child being institutionalized..."

I was becoming more and more excited. If the single handicap of blindness could cause all this deprivation, what about the additional perceptual handicap of cerebral palsy? Wasn't Helen Keller an example of someone with a double handicap - deafness and blindness? Yet she had been able to learn with a good teacher.

Suddenly I was convinced that Rikki could learn. I felt more excited than I had for weeks. If the ability was there we were going to have to find it. Isn't this the key role of occupational therapy to look for ability in spite of disability?

The way suddenly became crystal clear. My job was to teach skills of daily living and community adjustment, and I was not going to be either threatened or coerced away from doing my job just because the patient was different from the others. But the right road is not always the smoothest and the next day something happened that widened the gap between the two factions of the staff and I was to find myself caught firmly in the middle.

Chapter 4

A MATTER OF UNDERSTANDING

"People accustomed from infancy to lie down on Down feathers have no idea how hard a paving-stone is, without trying it."
Charles Dickens "Hard Times"

The next morning I arrived on Rikki's ward at the usual time for her treatment, but she was not there.

"Where's Rikki?" I asked the ward clerk.

"A porter came for her about fifteen minutes ago," she said. "I thought she'd gone to O.T. Let's look at the board."

A large time-table was posted on the wall of the ward office with coloured tickets indicating the different disciplines for every hour of the day for each patient. Two tickets had been inserted beside Rikki's name for eight-thirty: psychology in addition to occupational therapy.

"Of all the nerve!" I exclaimed. "That's my time. And they didn't even ask!"

I was annoyed. It was always understood that each discipline would inform the other if times had to be changed. I arranged to see another patient instead of Rikki, and I had just returned to my department when I heard my name being called on the intercom.

"Miss Wallace, please call switchboard. Miss Wallace, please call switchboard."

I picked up the telephone and dialed the operator.

"Yes, Miss Wallace. Please call Miss Robertson in psychology immediately."

I dialed psychology and was put through to the lab.

"This is the psychometrist speaking. We have a patient here called Erika Chase. We're having a little trouble. She's become quite hysterical and keeps screaming for you. I can't get her to stop. Can you come over?"

I hung up the telephone. Rikki's chart had noted that there had been tantrums in the past, but she'd been completely happy and cooperative since she'd come to Rehab. I wondered what had happened.

Rikki was still sobbing, her face streaked with tears, when I arrived.

"I'm sorry," she sobbed. "I'm sorry Sally. I've caused so much trouble. Don't be angry."

"Rikki, why should I be angry?" I replied. "Now come along and we'll go back to the O.T. ward. We'll go the long way around outside in the sunshine and you can tell me all about it."

Rikki was silent for the next ten minutes while I pushed her wheelchair away from the psychology building and out to the paths and lawns that surrounded the various buildings of the complex. Back in the treatment clinic I found a corner in the O.T. Quiet Workshop and gave her a wet towel to wipe her face.

"Someone came and took me away," she said. "It was a porter I think, but he didn't speak English and I couldn't understand him. He took me down in the elevator to an underground place. I could hear the pipes and heaters and I got more and more frightened. Then we came up again in another place. The lady asked me a lot of crazy questions, just going on and on. She asked me to tell her what colours were. She asked me to draw a picture, and I said I couldn't draw because I was blind. Then she asked me to draw shapes. She kept asking me the same question over and over and I kept telling her I couldn't see. But she didn't believe me. I said, "Didn't you hear me? I told you I was blind." Was she stupid or something? I told her over and over I couldn't draw anything."

She paused for a moment, wiping her wet face with her hand, and then continued, "I didn't understand some of the questions. I didn't know how to answer and I got more and more frightened about what would happen if I failed. Then she started to draw lines on the back of my hand, and that's when something just snapped. "Sally, I couldn't help it. I started to scream. I just... just... couldn't."

She started to cry again.

"It's all right," I said. "It was only a psychology test. You didn't understand what was happening and the psychometrist didn't understand what it's like to be blind. It doesn't matter at all. Now you just settle down and I'll explain the whole thing to you. Later we'll go through that tunnel again. I don't suppose you ever knew that there are several buildings at this Rehab Centre, connected by a big underground tunnel."

How poorly we understand the world of the blind. How simple it would have been to explain to Rikki what the test was and where she was going, as one would to a child. And in order to administer a standardized test according to the rules, the same for all patients, to the extent of repeating the question three times, no allowance had been made for her blindness, or that she would be unable to perform the tasks that depended on vision. The results could not have been a true indication of her intelligence, particularly when she was in an emotional state close to terror.

The psychometrist could not have understood that she precipitated a startle response by trying to draw shapes on the back of Rikki's hand. She would not have known that a totally blind person lacks the ability to anticipate an action because she could not see it initiated. We all made mistakes with Rikki through our ignorance of blindness. I felt that I was only just beginning to understand how the world seemed to her, and how difficult it was for a sighted person to fully comprehend what it must be like to be born blind, to *never* have experienced a visual impression of anything. I was realizing how different this must be from becoming blind later in life.

The psychometrist was a technician trained to administer all standardized tests according to strict rules. The fault lay with us, the professionals, imposing our norms and our customs on a patient, without sufficiently understanding the whole person. But the day was not ruined for Rikki. She bounced back to her happy self again when she felt secure and a message that her new wheelchair had arrived at "Purchasing" cheered us both.

Rikki had been at Rehab for three weeks. I had one more week to teach her to transfer before the next conference, and this time I was determined that she should not know about the conference, because she always anticipated it with such anxiety.

Each day we worked on some aspect of telling the time with a Braille clock that I had obtained from the Agency for the Blind Gift Shop in Windford. One of my patients had made a little square wooden box to contain the clock, to make it easier to handle.

It's not easy to teach someone to tell the time when number concepts are weak. I tried to approach the problem as one would with a young child. I went over basic counting from one to twelve, establishing that Rikki had an idea of the quantities represented by each number and had not just learned them by rote, and explaining the function of the big and little hands. Rikki had learned to place the clock in the correct position with twelve at the top before beginning. Then she learned to locate the raised dots representing the numbers, and to count by fives.

In spite of this, she had still not grasped the idea. Each morning when I arrived I would say something like, "Rikki, how late am I to-day?" Then she would position and feel her clock and make an incorrect calculated guess.

"Wrong. You're guessing again," I would say, and we would repeat the process, going over and over where the big and little hands were, but still she had not grasped it.

"Why don't you understand, Rikki?" I would ask. "What am I missing? Have you heard the saying, if the student's not learning, the teacher's not teaching".

"One thing I don't understand," she said one morning, "is why the numbers sometimes have two names, like number eight, that is sometimes called twenty, but four is also called twenty."

I was pleased with her question because it indicated that she was learning to formulate logical questions to get information. This had been difficult for her. We talked about the hours and the minutes, and about what a pie looked like and how it could be cut into halves and quarters.

Sometimes when it seemed to be getting too complicated I would revert to some physical exercises instead, like bouncing on the bed beside her, counting bounces, or bouncing to music.

"You are funny," she laughed. "You want to do the craziest things!"

She did not understand that we were bouncing with a purpose. I was trying to teach her to shift her weight off her seat, preparatory to shifting from one place to another, called transferring. As soon as she had acquired enough balance I introduced another game that she found hilarious.

"Now don't be laughing too hard, Rikki." I cautioned, "or you'll fall right off the bed. I'm going to try to push you over and you must resist me. Come on now, don't fall. Resist me."

Leaning forward was most difficult because she was afraid of falling. She had to be held by the shoulders until she established her centre of balance. Once secure in trunk balance, she finally learned to draw one leg over the other knee. From there she was able to learn to take her shoes and socks off and feel her feet for the first time. This was such a triumphant achievement that tears of joy were rolling down her face.

"I never thought I would ever do this!" She sobbed.

For the rest of the week Rikki's progress continued more or less steadily. In the mornings we talked about radio programs, music and current affairs while we did the exercise routine, and she was finally able to do a side transfer with only a little assistance and the aid of a belt and a transfer board. The nursing staff was good about helping with eating skills at mealtime, so that she knew what she was eating and where everything was. She learned to use a short rocker knife to cut her meat; an adjustable plate-guard prevented food from sliding off the plate. She had to be taught to take small bites, and to eat more slowly. Years of eating defensively for fear her food would be stolen by other residents had taught her to eat as fast as possible, with complete disregard for table manners and this was unappetizing for anyone sitting opposite.

In the afternoons Rikki attended the "Heavy Workshop". She was given activities designed to improve muscle tone and coordination, and to teach missing concepts like "forward" and "back", "in front of" and "behind", "inside" and "outside". She learned to operate a stationary remedial bicycle with foot straps, variable resistance and mileage indicator so that her daily progress could be measured.

My case load was such that I could spend only one or two hours a day with Rikki. She always had an hour in physiotherapy, and the remainder of her day, apart from an afternoon rest period, was spent under the direction of a therapy assistant or in a recreational program.

One day Rikki was sanding a transfer board in the O.T. Heavy Workshop when she suddenly stopped work and said, "I have the strangest feeling that someone is watching me."

There was no one else in the workshop so I asked her who she thought was there.

"I think it's my father," she said. "I'm sure he's here. Would you look out in the hall?"

I went to the door. It was true that a man was standing in the hall watching Rikki as she worked. I asked him if he was looking for someone.

"That's my daughter, there," he said. "I just thought I'd come over and see how she's getting along, but I don't want to disturb anyone."

It was the first time I had met either of Rikki's parents. This man did have some resemblance to her in the colour of his hair and something about the line of his mouth but there the resemblance ended. He was a large man, with large hands and feet and a ruddy complexion, as though he worked outdoors. She was glad to "see" him and told him about all the exciting new things she was doing.

"Is that true?" he asked. "Is she really doing all these things? How come she never learned to do these things before, like when she was a child?"

I explained that Rikki needed trained people to teach her, and that it was only recently that therapists had the kind of training. I could see that she had a good relationship with her father. He teased her a lot, making fun of her hair hanging down over her eyes.

"How can we tell whether we're looking at the front or the back of her?" He asked, laughing.

I agreed that I thought she needed a haircut, but when this had been suggested by the nurses she had objected strenuously.

"I want to grow it long," she said.

I suggested that she might be able to look after her own hair if it were short. She agreed to think it over. After her father had left I asked her how she had known he was there. He had been completely silent.

"I knew," she said, "because he always uses that kind of shaving cream." I had not noticed any scent of shaving cream, but this taught me not to underestimate a blind person's ability to use the other senses more effectively than sighted people.

The next day the subject of hair-cutting was broached again by one of the nurses. Rikki remained adamantly against the idea until it was mentioned that it would mean a trip to the beauty salon in the shopping centre and a real hairdresser. This put the whole thing in a different perspective, and she agreed at once. The trip to the hairdresser was a great success and she was even invited to stay and have lunch with the hairdresser.

It was interesting to watch people's reaction to Rikki. She had the ability to put people at ease, but they frequently wanted to give her something. Blindness, in addition to confinement to a wheelchair, represented a devastating disability to most people. Their immediate reaction was thankfulness that this had not happened to them, followed by a pressing desire to make some gesture to help.

Rikki was acquiring an impressive collection of treasures, trinkets and bits of jewelry people had given her. The problem was that people who had gone out of their way to be kind would eventually find that they could no longer continue, and withdrew. She never saw that hairdresser again, but she was grateful to her for her kindness.

Her progress was astounding. I found it necessary to analyze her treatment program every day, so that we could aim at realistic small gains, leading to the desired goals, without imposing activities that were too demanding or boring. I tried to assure that each activity was meaningful to her, at times going through it myself with my eyes shut to determine the problems and the skills that were required. Her diligence never waned. She worked so hard, at times with the perspiration running down her face, that it was necessary to alternate strenuous work with intellectual demands. I was sure that she would have willingly continued to work all night. In spite of this, the element of fun was present too. I often tried to make a game of it, and there was lots of laughter and teasing.

Rikki's emotions were always close to the surface, so I learned not to take it too seriously when she over-reacted and laughed or cried too loud or too long. The offensive odor the physiotherapist had described was found to be caused by a certain medication. She had arrived with a bladder infection as well as a mild skin problem. When the medication was changed the odor and the skin problem disappeared.

One day I decided to use an in-house telephone to teach her to modulate her voice. It disturbed the other patients in the workshop and on the ward, and affected her relationship with other people. She had never been allowed to use a telephone, and regarded this as an exciting new skill. More important, it gave her immediate feedback, when I told her how far I had to hold the telephone from my ear when her voice was too loud.

I was disappointed and angry with the lack of interest of the Agency for the Blind. Repeated requests for help only produced the same result, they did not have the resources to help at this time. I had always thought of this Agency as the “umbrella” for all blind people, but now I was beginning to understand that they did not have the trained personnel to work with someone like Rikki. I felt sure, however, that they must have equipment that we could use. The Braille clock was already proving to be useful, and I wanted to try a “talking book” machine, so I decided to persevere to find out why they were being so evasive.

Chapter 5

NOTHING IS IMPOSSIBLE

"Believe and act as if it were impossible to fail."
Charles F. Kettering

As the day for the next conference drew nearer, Rikki became more and more disturbed. In spite of my hopes that she would not know about it, someone had told her and she was nervous and apprehensive.

"I don't want people talking about me behind my back." she said. "I want to know what they're saying."

Traditionally patients did not attend case conferences. Their presence tended to inhibit the reports and it was felt that knowledge of their complete diagnosis and medical details were not always in the best interest of all the patients. At the same time, I could understand Rikki's concern and the reasons why she wanted to be present.

"I cried all night, Sally," were her first words when I entered the ward.

As the nurses had not reported crying all night, I assumed that the crying was limited to the time Rikki was awake and that she had probably slept normally.

"I cry whenever I think of going back," she continued. "Are they really going to send me back next week? I won't be able to do any of these things when I go back there. Please tell them to let me stay."

The "Rehab" staff had been good to Rikki and she liked them. "They're the greatest," she would say. "I've never met so many good friends before in all my life. I just love everyone here."

She got along less well with the patients. They had their own problems and they were less tolerant of her incessant repetitive talking and exuberance.

"Why doesn't that lady in the next bed like it here?" She asked. "She says she hates physio and refuses to do her exercises. I told her she's lucky to be in such a nice place."

That day I had invited a field worker from the Agency for the Blind to come to lunch and to meet Rikki. Mr. Fielding, who was blind himself, arrived shortly before noon accompanied by his driver. As they walked along the corridor he showed me the correct way to guide a blind person by allowing him to take my arm and to walk slightly in front of him.

Mr. Fielding stopped briefly to fold his white cane and put it in his pocket. "We've been aware of Rikki since she was born," he said. "She has been registered, but you must understand that we're extremely limited in what we can offer someone so disabled, and it would not be possible for us to spare a field worker to go on any regular basis to an institution that is so far from the city".

"Not even if there were more there like her?" I asked.

He answered by explaining the services that they offered, such as an excellent prevention of blindness program, helping newly blinded persons to adjust to blindness, teaching Braille and providing training in Orientation and Mobility. There were some teachers of handicrafts such as leatherwork and basketry, but they did not have people skilled in teaching the kind of things that might be suitable for severely disabled people.

"Do you think your client would be interested in learning how to fold money?" He asked. "We fold the bills in different ways so that we can tell them apart."

I explained that Rikki's needs were much more basic than that, and that she had never had any money of her own and would have to be taught money values before this would have any meaning for her. Rikki's greatest need now was language development and listening skills. I asked why it was so difficult for us to obtain a "talking book" machine. I had understood that these were supposed to be available to all blind persons.

"There's a big demand for them," he replied, "and they break down a lot. We haven't even got enough to supply our regular clients."

The luncheon meeting was disappointing. Mr. Fielding offered to have Rikki tested for Braille aptitude, which some of the "Rehab" team had thought was a good idea. Other than that he had no suggestions of how they could help. He promised to look into the "talking book" situation. It is as well that I didn't know that Rikki would wait three years for that machine.

Mr. Fielding departed after lunch and the case conference started soon after. Rikki's case was the first to be discussed.

Dr Pentland gave a brief review from the chart: "This nineteen year old female patient has now been with us for four weeks. It appears that she has made progress in occupational therapy, slight progress in physiotherapy and the social worker now expresses the view that the institutional placement is unsuitable. From the nursing point of view there have been gains on the ward. We seem to have no report from psychology. Why is there no report? This report was requested for to-day. Is someone here from that *illustrious* department?"

A young psychometrist, Joan Whitby, replied, "Yes, Dr. Pentland. Dr. Brough has asked me to report that the patient was uncooperative and he recommends a more complete neuro-psychology testing."

Dr Pentland sighed. "Very well. May we hear the O.T. report please?"

I began to read: "This patient continues to progress daily. The new wheelchair arrived and has enabled us to teach Rikki to transfer to and from the bed and the toilet. She can now undress herself, including her shoes and socks, and she can now reach her feet for the first time. She can't dress herself yet because she lacks sufficient position sense to arrange her clothing, but I think she's going to be able to learn this. Her voice is becoming more pleasant and she's learning to feed herself.

"This patient is very resistant to going back to the institution." I continued. "She's afraid that if she goes back she'll lose all the skills she has gained."

"She's right. She will," said Dr. Pentland. "I think the time has come to invite the staff from the institution to meet with us for a special conference, so they can be shown in detail how to manage this young woman. They must be shown what she can do and how to care for her. May we have the social service report, please?"

Judy Dance had been seeing Rikki on a daily basis, and had met with her family as well as with the social worker, Philip Martin, from the institution.

"There's a possibility of a suitable placement for Rikki near Stemler," Judy said. "Her parents and the institution have agreed to let us submit an application. It's called Palmer House, and is designed for young people with cerebral palsy. The only problem is that they may not accept blind people.

"The only other alternative to the institution is a nursing home, and they've all refused to consider someone who is blind as well as wheelchair dependent. One home for chronic care refused because Rikki is too young. All their patients are terminally ill and elderly -- not a suitable placement for a young girl."

"What role is the Agency for the Blind playing in all this?" asked Dr. Pentland.

"The O.T. and I met with them," replied Judy, "and they said they had nothing useful to offer. They couldn't even promise equipment like a "talking book" machine. They don't seem to have resources for multiply handicapped people."

"Is there any more discussion on this case?" asked the doctor.

"Yes," I replied. "I'm wondering why there's never been a vision test for this patient. There's no record of one on the chart."

Dr. Pentland thumbed through the chart, turning the pages rapidly back and forth. "The diagnosis is retrolental fibroplasia. You are right that there are no details about the eye condition, and there is no record of this patient ever having been examined by an ophthalmologist."

"Can anything be done to restore the vision?" I asked.

Dr. Pentland did not reply. Turning to the ward nurse who was taking the minutes he said, "You will arrange with the Memorial Hospital to have a complete ophthalmologic examination done as soon as possible. You will set up an appointment for a neuro-psychology test to be done as well, *we hope before the patient has left.* The social service department will arrange for the staff of the Maplegrove institution to meet with us here for a special conference."

He closed the file. "What is the opinion of this conference? I suggest a three-week extension of this patient's assessment period, with discharge arranged for three weeks from to-day. Agreed? Next patient please."

Several staff members joined me as we left the conference room. We walked together along the corridor, past the ward office towards the elevator.

"So we've got a three week reprieve, Sally," said Judy. "Would you like to work with me to try to find some place that will take Rikki, in case Palmer House falls through?"

"Yes, of course, Judy," I replied. "I wonder if there has ever been a vision test done." The state of the art in ophthalmology has changed a lot in twenty years. Maybe something could be done surgically. That would entirely change Rikki's Rehab potential. We've got to find some place for her so that she doesn't go back to that institution. Have you got any ideas, Judy? How can I help?"

"There's one other possibility, Sally," said Judy. "Have you ever heard of the Cheshire Homes Foundation?"

"Yes, I do remember hearing something about it, but I've forgotten what it was. Is it some sort of religious organization, Judy?"

"No, I think it was started in England for paraplegics after the war. There are several in this country as well as in Europe and India. They may not have support services during the daytime, but I'm going to find out."

"Sounds worth investigating. I don't blame Rikki at all for not wanting to go back," I said. "She sees this as her first big chance to get out of the institution. There must be some place where she could go."

"Yes, and I think you're absolutely right about her not being retarded. Pity about the psych test. You'd think they, of all people, would have shown more interest and understanding. Are you coming down in the elevator?"

"No. I think I'll pop along to the ward ...tell her she's got another three weeks. She'll want to know. I'll be glad to help all I can Judy. Just call me."

Rikki was sitting in her usual position, with her head dropped forward, listening to the thin whine of her little portable radio.

"Hi Rikki," I said. "Guess what! Good news. We've got another three weeks. But that is final, so we'll have to work extra hard. Tomorrow we start dressing techniques in the morning and some special games in the afternoon."

The inevitable flood of tears began to roll down Rikki's cheeks again.

"Hey now, that's not the way to greet good news. Don't you want to stay?" I laughed.

"I sure do, Sally," she replied. "I sure do. Now I don't have to worry for three more weeks. And Sally, may I ask you something about animals -- like what horses and dogs and cows are really like? Do you think I could ever sit on a horse?"

I laughed. "Good grief, Rikki, what an idea! Nothing's impossible. We'll think about it. Whatever made you think of getting on a horse?"

"Dan Adams, the recreation director. He told me that sometimes handicapped people can get on horses. And we've been reading about animals and I'd like to really know what they're like."

"You're right Rikki that disabled people can often ride horses, but they have to be taught in a very controlled way, with very gentle, obedient horses. Helpers usually walk along beside the rider while someone leads the horse. I don't think there's a program like this in this city, but maybe Dan knows of one."

"Dan said he does know of a place where I could maybe just get on a horse -- not really ride, you know - just to see what it's like. I've never seen a horse, and if you helped..."

I promised to talk to Dan. "You do give me the toughest assignments, Rikki."

I left the ward wondering if there might be some way we could give Rikki this experience before she had to leave. I didn't tell Rikki that I had been a rider myself. The horse would have to be very gentle, and the horses I knew would not have been suitable. Dan must have a stable in mind if he suggested it.

I had learned so much working with this patient, but perhaps the most important thing was never to say anything was impossible. I had also learned the importance of gaining the complete trust of my patients by never promising anything I could not fulfill. I took each day as it came, never trying to predict the result until I tried, and each day had seen a new achievement of some sort. Now Dan and I were going to have to find a quiet horse.

Chapter 6

TRY, TRY AGAIN

"Faith is believing in things when common sense tells you not to."
George Seaton

One morning, I arrived on Rikki's ward quite early to work on dressing techniques. Undressing was easy for Rikki now, but dressing was more difficult because it involved positioning of the clothing, something Rikki had never learned. An additional problem, frequently experienced by people with cerebral palsy, was an impaired sense of touch and joint position, so these skills had to be taught and did not come naturally.

Rikki was sitting in her wheelchair in her nightgown, listening to her radio. Ample green curtains were drawn around the other three beds to provide privacy for dressing. The heat wave had finally spent itself and the cool crisp morning air gave everyone more energy. Rikki looked particularly eager as I announced my arrival with my usual greeting.

"I heard you coming off the elevator, Sally," said Rikki. "I'd know your step anywhere. But guess what!

I've got some great news for you. I bet you won't guess what has happened."

"You won the lottery?" I exclaimed, laughing.

"No, but now I can tell the time. Where's that clock? Here it is. Now....it's exactly fifteen minutes past eight and you're fifteen minutes early. How about that? I now *know* what the hands are saying. I'll never make a mistake again."

"Why, that's marvelous, Rikki! What happened? How did you suddenly catch on?"

"You want to know what it was?" She asked with enthusiasm. "I never really understood what you meant by "before" and "after" the hour -- the twelve that is. I learned what "front" and "back" means, and "in front of" and "behind", but I didn't get it, 'til suddenly, whammo, I got the idea. It just came to me. Now I don't think I'll ever make a mistake because I understand all the positions."

It was true. I moved the hands to different positions and she got them all right for the first time after five weeks. This was a real break-through, like Helen Keller finally connecting the word "water" with something wet -- the concept that a word could represent a reality. It was finally through a spatial concept that Rikki had learned how two little pointers on a clock face could represent all the hours, minutes and seconds of the day.

It was not just the sense of achievement that excited me so much, but the solving of a conceptual problem. But for Rikki, this achievement gave her the experience of winning, of victory, of success over something that was previously unknown to her, and it proved that we were winning, that she *could* learn these things, that I was on the right track.

"That is simply super, Rikki," I said. "That is the very best news you could have given me. Now let's get on with the dressing, and see if you can learn that too, because it involves similar problems."

Dressing techniques had to be broken down into basic step-by-step procedures. This time we were concentrating on a pullover sweater. I handed it to Rikki and she dropped it in her lap. As I watched, she proceeded to tumble it around, like a piece of clothing in an automatic dryer. It was tempting to reach over and help her, but I waited and watched her for several minutes.

"What are you doing, Rikki?" I asked quietly.

"I'm going to put on my sweater."

I waited a few more minutes. The movements became more and more hurried, until the sweater finally fell to the floor. Rikki was silent. "Where is the sweater now, Rikki?"

"It's gone."

"Where has it gone?"

"I don't know. The trouble is, Sally, that it didn't make a noise. It just disappeared."

I thought about the quotation about voices disappearing into nothingness. Of course. This is what happened. "OK Rikki. I understand. But the sweater has to weigh something, so when you let go, it just dropped. It was too light to make a noise, but it has to be on the floor. Do you know what gravity is?"

"Not really. Why is it on the floor? Where exactly *is* the floor?"

Then I realized that there was a deficit here too. Was it the concept of "down", or was it a lack of understanding of the principle of gravity? What's a good definition of a floor? I explained this as briefly as I could and picked up the sweater. I would have to get something to explain the principle of gravity, but for now I decided to continue with the dressing.

"O.K. Rikki, it's not going to work like that, is it? We need a system. Now, all garments have parts to them. There's the part that covers the front of your chest, the part that covers the back, and the sleeves. There's an inside and an outside, a neck part and a waist part. Now, let's see if you can find these parts of the sweater."

Again, as I had done so often before when working with Rikki, I closed my eyes so that I could see the problem as it would seem to her. She had to learn what a seam felt like, then the ribbing around the waist and cuffs, and then find the label at the back of the neck.

"The label is always at the back of the neck on the inside."

"Why? Why does it have to be there?"

"I suppose because it is least likely to show there. The label identifies the maker of the garment, but the person who wears it doesn't want people to see that, and it helps the person wearing it to tell quickly which is the back and which is the front. The back usually comes up higher in the neck, so the sweater wouldn't feel comfortable if you put it on back to front. Can you understand all this, Rikki?"

"Yes, but what do you mean by the inside? Why does it matter which side of the sweater is on the outside?"

"Because the knitting looks unfinished on the inside of a sweater, and not as nice as the outside. Also, when it's sewn together there's usually a seam on the inside that's not supposed to show. So you have to feel carefully to make sure that the seams are on the inside. Now, try to find the seams on this sweater. Can you tell where they are?"

"This sure is complicated," said Rikki.

"Right. Now find the label. Good. Now lay the sweater on your lap so that the side with the label on it is on top and the waistband is against your tummy... Now grab that back waistband and pull it over your head."

It was tempting to reach over and help her, but the only way she was going to learn was from my verbal instruction, because she couldn't see my actions, and the hard thing for me was to put those actions into words so that she could understand. I was interested to see that, while her right arm was spastic and usually resting in a flexed position, she was able to use her limited grasp to assist her good arm.

"It works," cried Rikki. "I can do this! Why didn't anyone ever tell me things like this?"

Progress was slow but steady. Every day we went over the routine with each garment, practicing a sequence that never changed, and each day a few mistakes sent Rikki into a panic when she lost her place. But gradually she began to understand.

Rikki's days were quite full now, and it had become even more important to arrange her time-table so she was not overloaded and would not be too tired for her physiotherapy and frequent counseling with her social worker. In addition, every afternoon a teacher came from the Agency to assess her aptitude for Braille. I knew that Rikki had impaired tactile discrimination in her fingers, and that Braille was probably not in the picture for her, but she had made such positive gains that the treatment team wanted the opinion of a qualified teacher. As I suspected, even the larger version of Braille dots proved to be too difficult for her to identify, and the lessons were discontinued.

When Rikki had been at Rehab for six weeks a group of five staff from the Maplegrove institution were invited to observe what she could do on the ward and then attend a case conference to discuss her present needs and her future placement back at the institution. They gathered around Rikki's bed to watch her transfer from bed to wheelchair, and to observe her dressing techniques and the special equipment that she was using.

All the Rehab staff working with Rikki were present at the conference that afternoon. Dr Pentland, as Chairman, presented the preliminary report: "This patient has made very significant progress during her six weeks with us," he concluded. "We would like to have your assurance that she will not regress when she returns to your facility."

"I'm not sure we can give you that." Said Mr. Blackstone, the senior member of the group. "You have to understand that we are not a rehabilitation centre. We have no facilities for the things you teach here."

"You have asked us to assess your patient," said Dr. Pentland. "You have asked us to tell you what she needs. She requires grab bars at the toilet and bath. She needs plate guards for her food. She needs to be allowed to transfer independently with a transfer board, with her bed the same height as her wheelchair. She needs exercise, and, above all, she needs education."

"I don't think they would allow any of that on the ward she's on," said Mr. Blackstone. "No one else does those things on that ward, and there are no bath tubs and no grab bars."

"Well then, she must be moved," said Dr. Pentland. "Do you have a more advanced ward?"

"Not really. There's a higher functioning ward, but it's not that high either. There are no bath tubs or grab bars on any of the wards, and besides, the staff on the other wards are not trained to deal with wheelchairs," said Mr. Blackstone.

"Nonsense, there's nothing to learning to work with wheelchairs. We will send a therapist out to instruct your staff on how to manage this patient. What about education? Do you have no educational facilities for these patients?"

This time one of the other counselors replied. "There is an Education Unit, but it's only for children. Rikki's too old to be placed there."

"But this girl is now starting to learn. Is there someone who could read to her? Are there books on the ward?"

"No books are allowed on the wards, Doctor. Books have to stay in the school, and besides, no one would have time to read to her. They're much too busy with the routine care."

Dr. Pentland looked through the file again. "Let me hear from the rest of you. What have you to say about this patient? We'll start with you, on my left."

Rikki was described as attention-seeking on the ward. "She sets herself above the others. She's not the only intelligent one there. There are many more like her."

"Where are these other intelligent patients?" Asked Dr. Pentland.

"Oh, they're all on different wards. They're not all in wheelchairs."

"Why is it so difficult to put this girl with other intelligent patients?"

"Because," said Mr. Blackstone, "you'd have to break down the barriers of the system to do that. Residents can't be moved from one ward or unit to another. It is against the rules."

"What about her equipment… her radio, her Braille clock, her tape recorder. Could she have these set up on the ward?" Asked Dr. Pentland.

"Not the way things are now. They'd all be broken in one day. These people are retarded, Doctor. Equipment like that has to be kept locked in the office, and there's no quiet place to use it. It would be quite impossible."

"Tell me something, Mr. Blackstone," said Dr. Pentland, "In your opinion, should this patient go back to your institution?"

"No. I don't think she belongs there at all."

The others seemed to agree. Another counselor added, "She's a disturber on the ward, Doctor. She's very demanding, and we have to treat them all the same. She can't have special privileges; it's not fair to the others. It's very unlikely that we could carry on with any of these programs."

The meeting was adjourned without anything being resolved, except that Rikki was to remain at least another two or three weeks, until a reply had been received from Palmer House.

Judy drew me aside as everyone got up to leave. "Stay behind a moment, Sally," she said. "We need a little mini conference, with just the four of us who've been working with Rikki." We sat down again after everyone had left.

"We can't let her go back to that place," said Judy. "She'd really think she'd failed, and she's done so well. What can we do?"

"I agree, Judy," I said. "There must be some alternative. And Rikki's not the only one here who needs a place to go."

"You're right," said Judy. "It's almost impossible for us to find suitable placements for some of our quadriplegics. Most of them have to go to nursing homes or chronic care hospitals. It's very discouraging. Just last week I took Peter Rondo over to a chronic hospital. He's only nineteen. They told him that they couldn't promise to get him dressed in time to go to college, and he wouldn't be able to play his music in the evening or have his friends in. He said he might as well be in jail. So his mother's going to hire an attendant for him and let him stay at home."

"That's terrible," said Carol, a physiotherapist. "Do you think there's any hope that Palmer House will take Rikki?"

"Not permanently, Carol," replied Judy. "But I think if we can get an assessment from them it might lead to something else. I'm hoping they'll take her for a three week assessment. The trouble is, they already have a long waiting list and we're not in their area. I'll phone them today."

"Have you found out anything more about Cheshire Homes? I asked.

"All I know is that someone in England started them for paraplegics. Most people's homes were not accessible for wheelchairs, so they all had to stay in hospitals. I'm trying to find out more about them. But Rikki would probably not be eligible because she's blind and because they don't seem to have daytime supervision."

We decided to enlist the help of all the staff and people from the community who might come, and hold a meeting to find out what would be involved in starting a home in the community. It would be a "brain-storming" meeting, some evening, as soon as possible, and Rikki's and Peter's parents would be invited.

I thought of something I'd read in the library a few days ago. It was the motto of the W. Ross Macdonald School for the Blind: "The Impossible is Only the Untried." Well, we had been working against all odds with Rikki, with many so-called impossible gains. We might as well continue as long as there were more impossible things that remained untried.

Chapter 7

AROUND THE BEND

"A single event can awaken within us a stranger totally unknown to us."
Antoine De Saint-Exupery

While the conference with the staff from the institution was anything but a success, it allowed another reprieve for Rikki. The following week it was decided unanimously that some different arrangements would have to be made if she were to be returned as planned to the institution. There had been a delay in the psychology testing and the Ophthalmologist's report had not yet been received. Rikki was still making progress in O.T., so it seemed advisable to delay discharge for another three weeks. Judy's telephone call to Palmer House was disappointing. They did occasionally take people in for assessment, but could not promise a space in the near future.

Every day I looked on the chart for the vision test. Finally I telephoned the Rehab records librarian. "According to the librarian at the Memorial Hospital where you say these tests were done," she said, "there is no record of this patient ever having been there. Are you absolutely certain that she went?"

"Of course she went," I replied. "I'm working directly with her, and I saw her going with one of the nurses. She told me about it after she returned. Besides, it's recorded on her chart."

"They have no record of this visit," she insisted. "The hospital is certain she could not have been there."

I decided to go immediately to Dr. Pentland. The only thing to do was to go right to the top, and Dr. Pentland could contact the ophthalmologist directly. Rikki was not the sort of person one would easily forget. I was totally unprepared for Dr. Pentland's reaction.

"Are you on some sort of crusade for this patient?" He charged angrily. "I don't like what I'm hearing. This woman is becoming much too attached to us. We're raising her expectations with nothing to offer her. I don't like your attitude… not at all! You're stirring up a lot of trouble. You were told when she came that she would go back there. That institution is full of people like her. You can't change the whole world. Just forget about her for awhile. Go off and do your job!"

Dr. Pentland had lost his temper. He was shouting, and I felt the colour rising in my face.

"Dr. Pentland," I replied, trying to control my voice. "This is an unjust situation. This girl has no clout, no one to go to bat for her, no influence. Is that why you don't want to help her? Are some patients more important than others? Doesn't she have as much right to treatment here as anyone else? Or is this place selective? Her whole future would change if she could see, yet you seem to attach no importance to even one vision test. This is pure and simple discrimination."

Dr. Pentland looked at me, his eyes half closed and full of anger. "Now you listen to me and listen well," he said. "This is a political situation that you know nothing whatever about and you stay out of it. It's none of your affair. You do your job and just keep your nose out of things that don't concern you."

By this time I had lost my nervousness. I was just plain angry. "Dr. Pentland," I said. "I'm a good therapist. I don't concern myself with political situations when it comes to patients, and I don't think politics have any place in medicine. My job is to help my patients to become as normal as possible. I'm not a technician who punches a clock. I'm a professional person, and I know my duty to my patients and this *does* concern me!"

Dr. Pentland picked up some papers from his desk. "You've made your point. I've made mine. You can go now."

The interview was over. I stopped in the doorway. "I'll go," I said, "but I'll say one more thing. If we don't receive that eye report by the end of next week I'm going to the press!" I walked out and closed the door.

I began to shake when I reached the elevator. I hated confrontations like this. I had always been the shy type. I didn't like Dr. Pentland, but that sort of thing never really became an issue in my work. Nobody ever likes everybody, and a professional person is usually above that sort of problem.

I wondered how someone like that could have become a doctor, someone so inhumane. Then I remembered one day in conference when he had stated that all health professionals were secretly sadistic, because they enjoyed their safe position of being healthy while their patients were not. Everyone had laughed at the time, taking it for a joke. Now I could see the truth of it - for him - certainly not for me. I'd become a therapist because I wanted to help people to enjoy life as I did, never because I enjoyed seeing them sick or helpless.

In any large organization, no matter how clever or competent the staff may be, we are always dealing with personalities. No two people are ever alike, in training, experience, competence or in personality and Dr. Pentland was certainly different in personality. It comes out in different ways and much of it is play-acting, portraying oneself in a certain role.

Dr. Pentland, coming in as he did like a "new broom", demonstrated a large ego from the start, essentially establishing the pecking order, and his initial methods, while irritating, insulting and intimidating at times, kept us all on our toes and positively produced the best treatment services this clinic had ever offered.

He had hardly been here three weeks before he began to change the status quo. First it was our traditional green uniforms that had to go in favour of hospital white lab coats, to be worn over regular street clothes, to give a more professional hospital appearance.

The next areas to be attacked were our "workshops", now to be called treatment rooms. Out went the weaving looms and archaic printing press and in came a model kitchen, a clerical centre with typewriters and business equipment, standardized performance tests, and simulated work areas with equipment to promote carefully prescribed and graded skills training.

Home visits were expected where indicated to assure safety and independence upon discharge. Workplace visits helped us to simulate a patient's work environment. Finally, all therapists were now required to write daily progress reports directly on the patients' ward files.

The personalities of patients were of course affected by their health problems. This was understood, Rikki tended to over-react to everything. She could break into tears at the slightest provocation, and turn it all off just as quickly.

I took the elevator to the third floor and tried to pull myself together. The entire Rehab Centre knew Rikki by now, from the cleaning staff and porters to the office clerks and secretaries, as well as the medical staff. Their attitude to her ranged from admiration, pity or amusement to hostility, dislike and even anger. Rikki left nobody passive. Like it or not, no one who met Rikki could help thinking "What would I do if I were in her shoes?"

It's interesting to see how pity takes on so many disguises. It sometimes makes people over-friendly, so that they talk down, the way some people alter their voices when talking to a child or a little dog. Some would give Rikki small gifts, as though atoning for their own guilt, making it up to her in some way, and then rationalizing and silently withdrawing when they ran out of resources or could not keep up the pace.

I learned early that it was impossible to fool an intelligent blind person. They always knew. Yet people would continually underestimate Rikki's intelligence and attempt to deceive her by being less than truthful. She always saw through this but she never held it against anyone, enjoying the gesture while it lasted, as with the hairdresser.

Rikki was singing as I stepped off the elevator and walked towards her ward. She had a strong, clear treble voice, much like a boy soprano, and right on key. "Edelweiss, edelweiss, and every morning you greet me..." She seemed unaware of the small audience of patients that had drawn near to hear her, some in wheelchairs, one on crutches, enjoying the singing, but not joining in. I stood by the doorway and listened.

"...Bless my homeland forever." And then, "Hi Sally. I knew you were there. I watched "The Sound of Music" last night."

"You *watched*?" I asked. "How can you watch when you can't see, Rikki?"

"I watch my way and you watch yours. Was it ever a good show. I liked it."

"Did you understand it, Rikki?"

"Yes, I did, except for one thing. Why did the family, you know, the mother and father and all that, have to leave their home and climb up the mountain? What was wrong with the place where they lived? What were they so afraid of?"

As I explained the Nazi invasion of Austria and the Second World War to Rikki, I realized that she knew nothing of the war and that all the signs of war in that film, the goose-stepping, swastikas, Nazi flags, military uniforms, were all visual background, and not a prominent part of the dialogue. Her interpretation was otherwise not significantly different from the description a sighted person might have given. She was able to describe the time of year, the characters, the music, and she really had understood the story and enjoyed it. This was to be the first of many times when I became aware that visual acuity is only one component of vision, and that blind people could develop amazing compensating skills by using the senses of hearing, smell, and touch more acutely than a sighted person.

Each day started with some exercise routine, designed for strengthening and balance, as well as body awareness and increased range of motion, and each day saw new gains. From balancing on the bed and establishing her "righting" reflex, we had progressed to standing with assistance, just enough to do a pivot transfer and sit down again in a different place. In this way, Rikki was able to learn to transfer from bed to chair, then chair to chair, and, finally, to Rikki's complete amazement and delight, from wheelchair to toilet.

The ultimate transfer took place, however, one afternoon when Dan and I were able to take the last hour of the day off to visit a near-by stable and try to put Rikki up on a horse.

I wheeled her out to the clinic parking lot. Once positioned correctly beside the passenger seat, she placed her transfer board to bridge the gap between the car and her wheelchair, as she'd been taught. She then slid quite easily across the board into the front passenger seat. I put the seat cushion, arm rests and foot rests into the back seat, while Dan lifted the wheelchair into the trunk. Twenty minutes later we were guiding Rikki through the doorway into the stable.

It was an old-fashioned little stable with a concrete floor, and sheltering not more than ten thoroughbred hunter-jumpers. Bob McLeod, the stable manager, led out Gunga Din, the biggest horse but also the quietest, until he was standing obediently beside the grain bin. The other horses nickered and shuffled in their stalls, acknowledging the company. The stable was clean, but smelled distinctly of hay and manure, and Rikki loved every minute of it.

"Now don't you worry, Sally. Don't you be nervous for me. I'm not nervous at all. I'll be O.K. You'll see. Let me see you, Gunga old boy. Come to me Gunga."

Quietly I said to Dan, "How are we going to do this, Dan? Do you think if we could get her up on the grain bin we could transfer her over from there?"

Together we worked out a method. We moved Rikki from the grain bin over to the horse's back in a side-saddle position, then helped her to lift her right leg across over the withers to the other side. It worked. There was Rikki, higher than any of us, up on the horse's back, seventeen hands high. Good old Gunga Din didn't bat an eye or twitch a whisker.

Rikki passed her left hand slowly over the smooth hide, mane to shoulder, feeling the texture and the warmth of the animal. As Dan and I held her securely on each side, Bob led the horse forward at a slow walk, the large hoofs smacking the concrete floor in a rhythmic cadence.

"*Now* I know what that sound is they call 'clippity clop!'" exclaimed Rikki. "It's his feet! I always thought it was his teeth."

After Rikki returned to her wheelchair the horse willingly lowered his head so that she could feel his ears.

"What's *that*?" she asked. "An ear?... Really?... It's not like my ear."

When Rikki was back in her wheelchair Bob held a hoof so that she could feel it, and explained how horses were shod, where they lived and what they ate.

The visit to the stable was not only the highlight of the week for Rikki, but it became a focal point to work from because it generated thought and conversation outside herself. But her endless repetitive chatter about her own achievements had become boring in the extreme to both residents and staff. There was not one person there who was not trying to achieve some private personal goal, in some cases sheer survival, and Rikki's untiring energy, vigour, hard work, and crowing over every success was tolerated but tiresome, particularly because so many of her achievements were things that everyone else took for granted. Yet few spoke rudely to her. They were able to relate much more easily to the cerebral palsy condition than to the blindness. Most felt that blindness was a devastating disability and thought it a miracle that a blind person could do anything at all.

There is no doubt that many thought that Dan and I had gone completely 'round the bend when Rikki told them that she had been riding a real horse, and she enjoyed their reaction. In truth, they were genuinely impressed, and the change in their attitude to her was not missed by Rikki.

As the time approached for her discharge, Rikki again became more and more nervous on the ward, and the old behavior problems began to appear again. Then several things happened at the last minute to cause another delay. A telephone call from the institution informed us that, due to a case of hepatitis on the Unit, they would be unable to accept her back for two more weeks. Dr. Pentland was away on leave, also for two weeks. The team met briefly and decided that Rikki's discharge would have to be delayed until the institution was able to accept her.

Chapter 8

PROVIDING A LINK

"The world is round and the place which may seem like the end may also be only the beginning."
Ivy Baker Priest, "Parade"

In wondering how to use the next two weeks to the best advantage, and knowing that they would certainly be the last at Rehab for Rikki, I decided to introduce a new element into the training program.

A treatment centre specializing in rehabilitation and physical medicine would be expected to concentrate its main efforts on the physical needs of the patient, but I was beginning to suspect that true rehabilitation for some patients might not be physical. In Rikki's case, during the past ten weeks, we had been successful in teaching her basic self-help skills using physical or what was called functional restoration techniques, but with only limited results as far as mobility was concerned. While she had learned to do a pivot transfer, to dress and feed herself and to tell the time, and had gained some useful function in her right hand, she had reached a plateau physically. It now occurred to me that she still had a potential to improve mentally. We were not going to cure the cerebral palsy or the blindness, but her mind was the one part of her body that showed a good prognosis for more development.

It is hard to imagine the affect of a severely limited environment on the human mind, and if the body is equally restricted by immobility, abnormal living conditions, lack of stimulation and no contact with the real world, this is bound to delay mental development and behavior.

Rikki had not even had access to books that could have been her windows into the normal world and could have provided not only knowledge, but companionship and language. Are eyes the windows of the soul, or is it language? In Rikki's case, it might be language, because, as her ability to comprehend words and use them increased, so did her thought patterns, ideas, and learning ability. This then should be the next step in her rehabilitation.

I had made several home visits to Rikki's parents, to keep them informed of her progress and to suggest ways that they could help, as well as to gain insight into the home needs and life-style for the occasional times when they were able to have her at home. They had been cooperative, although skeptical, and wanted to be included, so I made a point of contacting them regularly with reports of Rikki's progress. They reacted with a mixture of incredulity and pleasure that Rikki was doing so well, but not without an element of anger and resentment that all this had not happened much earlier.

For this reason I did not feel it would be amiss to ask the parents to purchase a portable cassette tape recorder for Rikki. As expected, they were pleased to be asked and supplied it immediately.

Putting the cassette cartridge into the tape recorder presented the next challenge. She approached the problem the same way she had dealt with the pullover, by trial and error, without comprehending the spatial principles involved. I finally used Lego building bricks and let Rikki help to build a structure with four walls and a roof, with a doorway large enough for her hand. When she understood this particular concept of "inside" and "outside" that was different from the pullover she was able to apply it to the tape recorder with immediate success.

Learning to press individual keys presented no real problem, but having to press two keys together in order to record our voices was more difficult and took some practice.

Hearing her own voice for the first time, Rikki did not recognize it as her own. Then there was embarrassment, but before long she became intrigued by how she could alter her voice to show expression, tone or pitch, or to imitate someone else. She was particularly pleased to hear her own singing voice and to hear that it was good.

One day I took Rikki to a shopping centre. We wheeled in and out of all sorts of stores, learning about how books, clothing, shoes, candy, baked goods and perfumes were sold. Rikki enjoyed trying to guess what sort of store it was from the scent. She was impressed by the great quantities of merchandise and by the rows and rows of books.

"I had no idea there were so many books," she said, as she trailed the back of her hand along the shelves. "Tell me the names, Sally. What are they all about?"

We talked about fiction, mystery, adventure, history, geography, travel, religion and finally biography.

"What kind of people have biographies written about them," Rikki asked.

"Let's look," I suggested. "Here is one about the Trapp Family Singers... that was the "Sound of Music" family. Here's one about a hockey player, and another about a famous doctor, Dr Grenfell. Here's one Rikki, which you might recognize. It's the story of Lawrence Welk."

"Oh Sally, I just love the Lawrence Welk Show. Do you think they would lend us that one to read?"

"This is a store, Rikki, not a library where you can borrow books. We'll go to a library another time. But if you'd like to buy this book we can see if we have enough money. It's a paper-back and doesn't cost as much as the hard-cover books."

"I'd like to do that," said Rikki. "We could read it on tape, so I could read over and over. How much money do we need?"

I gave her some money, counting it out carefully, and told her how to hold it up to the cashier and to wait for some change. We talked about the relative costs of things as we went along. The visit was a success.

Rikki was able to identify with the young Lawrence Welk, who wanted so desperately to learn to play the accordion, but her attention waned as we got deeper into the book, with discussions about legal contracts and one-night-stands across the United States continent, so I found it necessary to be selective in my reading to hold her attention. Her limited vocabulary made it difficult for her to fully understand an entire paragraph without some additional explanation. If not challenged at regular intervals about the story, a misunderstood word might send her off into a day-dream.

The tapes served another purpose. They allowed Rikki to go over the material again. She enjoyed hearing her own voice on the recording along with mine, and this helped to hold her attention. At first there was hardly a sentence that she understood entirely because many words represented objects that she had never seen. For example, she didn't know what a coconut was except that it was something used in desserts for flavour. She asked if it grew already shredded on bushes. One day she asked if pineapple grew with the hole already in the middle, or why it always had a hole in the middle like a doughnut. In each case, I brought in the actual fruit, cut it open, and let her feel and taste it.

Soon Rikki had so many tapes that it became necessary to distinguish one from the other, so I devised a form of raised dot labeling simpler than Braille. It was obvious that she was unlikely ever to develop enough tactile discrimination to read Braille for pleasure, but she was able to use this modified version to identify her tapes. It was obvious now that she would have to develop much better language comprehension skills before she would benefit from "Talking Books", so I decided to try to work on this in the time we had left.

Gerald Durrell's "My Family and Other Animals" followed Lawrence Welk and was an immediate success. Rikki enjoyed the reading sessions, but these were taking a lot of time. I was now doing the recording in my own time at home, usually an hour or so every night, as well as preparing questions on each chapter, so I could tell how much she had understood. During the day she would listen to the chapter by herself, sometimes several times, before trying to answer the questions.

She was able to identify with every one of that delightful family, and was as fascinated with Durrell's descriptions of the small creatures of the insect world as anyone discovering creatures for the first time under a microscope.

"I can hardly wait for the next chapter," she would say.

But Rikki was not the only one who was learning and improving. Listening to my own reading as well as her response, helped me to learn to read clearly but informally, interrupting it with short explanations or abrupt questions, to assure all along that she was still following and not off in a day-dream or needing to ask a question. Sometimes I couldn't help laughing and Rikki would say, "What's funny?" As I stopped to explain, I realized that she had never developed a sense of humour. I wondered at what stage of mental development this occurred, or if it ever occurred in a person who was truly mentally delayed.

Does a baby learn to think when he begins to acquire language? What role do words play in thinking, the ability to visualize, to express emotion, and to conceptualize? How do congenitally blind people dream without language skills?

One day I was so absorbed in my reading that I'd forgotten about Rikki. Then I realized that she had fallen asleep in her wheelchair. I reached over and pushed the "stop" button on the recorder. It made a sharp click sound and she woke up with a start.

"You must be tired, Rikki."

"Oh no, Sally, not tired. Please keep on reading."

"What was I reading about, Rikki?"... Silence. "Well, I'll just take you back to the ward so you can have a rest."

"No! No! Please Sally," pleaded Rikki. "I promise. I won't go to sleep again."

There were loud wails and crying all the way back and heads turned towards us to see what was happening, but back we went. I felt mean because it had been my fault more than Rikki's, but this was an opportunity to force Rikki to improve her attention span. Rikki had never had this sort of discipline imposed upon her. She never fell asleep again in a reading session and her listening skills improved daily.

Rikki had now been with us for twelve weeks. As the inevitable day of discharge approached, she became more and more depressed and difficult on the ward. She begged everyone to find her a place to go, anything at all instead of going back to the institution. There was not one patient or member of staff who was unaware of the plight of this girl, but they were firmly divided according to their own feelings as to whether she should go back or not. Some felt that it would be a relief when she left so we could all get back to a normal routine.

At ten o'clock on the appointed day I went up to Rikki's ward. She was sitting in her wheelchair surrounded by brown paper shopping bags stuffed with her clothes and possessions. Much of her clothing had never been unpacked.

On her lap was her much-prized tape recorder. A cardboard box on the floor beside the bed contained her new equipment; plate guard, special meat knife, transfer belt, wooden box containing her cassette tapes, exercise equipment, little radio, oddments of souvenirs from the many people she had met, and Braille clock in its special box. Rikki's face was wet with tears, her nose running, her voice constricted with sobs. It was a dramatic moment, and she played it out without restraint, sobbing that she would never forget us, no matter what happened to her, and that someday she would come back.

"Rikki," I said. "There's something about me you don't know."

Rikki's sobs stopped. "What Sally?" She said.

"I never say good-bye, Rikki."

"You don't?" She asked. "Good. Then we don't have to. But when will I ever see you again?" The sobs started all over again.

It was then that I suggested my idea. "You've enjoyed the reading we've been doing, haven't you? What would you think of continuing the reading by mail? I would send you a tape to read and you would send me a reply."

"Yes, I'd really like to do that. If only I could hear your voice I wouldn't be so lonely."

"It's settled then. Next week I'll send you a cassette tape. But only on one condition, Rikki. I'll only send tapes in reply to yours. When you reply to mine and tell me what you thought of the story I'll send you another, but if you stop replying, so will I."

"It's a deal," she said. "It's a great idea."

This would provide a link for her with this new world she had discovered and was so reluctant to leave, and would somehow help her to feel that she had achieved something useful and that she had not totally failed.

"It's all right now, Sally," she said, for all the world like someone going to her execution, "I'm ready. Will you come with me to the car? And please see that they let me do the car transfer myself."

"Of course," I laughed. "You don't think you're going to get away without making a perfect transfer on your last day, do you?"

We went down in the elevator, Rikki calling everyone by name as she went. "Good-bye Tanya, Gerry, Mark, Marg and Phyllis," all of whom she had come to know better than I did. "Don't forget me, will you? Don't do anything I wouldn't do."

A large black limousine with uniformed chauffeur stood in the parapet, the Government insignia on its door. Rikki's possessions were tossed into the back seat. Then the chauffeur bent over, picked her up, and swiftly placed her in the back seat beside her luggage, before she had a chance to tell him that she wished to do the transfer by herself.

"You see, Sally? They won't let me do anything. Where's my transfer belt? Will my new wheelchair fit in? Did we remember all the parts?"

As the car drove off the last I saw of Rikki was the small round figure, head bent forward, looking for all the world exactly as she had looked when I first saw her. Slowly I walked back into the darkened hallway, where no one could see that my eyes were wet.

PART 2--THE LETTERS

"There is no thought without words."
John Dewey

We missed Rikki -- not all in the same way, but we were all aware of a change after she had left. In retrospect it occurred to me how important it was to treat the whole person. What was the use of teaching mobility, transfer and dressing skills that were not likely to be used after discharge? In those past twelve weeks how much had we given that young girl that was useful to her? At least thirty-three medical professionals had interviewed or tested Rikki and each had placed a report on her chart, but how many of us had given her anything of lasting value?

The neuro-psychology report did not appear on the chart until after she had left, and it merely indicated that she was unable to complete most of the test. The prognosis for further learning was "guarded". In fact, it was two months after she had left when we finally received the ophthalmology report, with apologies that the report had been mislaid by a medical intern. The condition was described as permanent congenital blindness. The patient was described as alert and intelligent.

I had suggested the idea of corresponding by cassette tape just before Rikki left, partly to allay a scene at the time of departure, but mainly because I felt that she deserved at least some link with this new world that she had discovered and was so reluctant to leave.

I decided to make the messages as impersonal as possible to encourage Rikki to talk about the story and subjects outside herself. I would continue with Gerald

Durrell's "My Family and Other Animals", but I did not expect the tape exchange to go on for long after she had re-adjusted to life in the institution. I put my first cassette in the mail the next day.

Rikki surprised me - again. She continued to send messages on a regular basis in reply to my stories and questions. A school teacher who was employed at the institution through the Board of Education, agreed to allow Rikki to go to the schoolroom on a daily basis to listen to the stories I had sent, and helped her to send the replies. It would have been impossible for her to do this on the ward.

More than one hundred cassette audio tapes were exchanged over a period of a year and a half. Only a representative number are included here, as many are repetitive. During that time I was interested to see how her communication skills were changing, her struggle with simple semantics, her favourite phrases, like "nobody ever told me", her concern not to offend, were all evident from the tapes. But to me, the most exciting development was how her increasing understanding of language was accompanied by a thirst for knowledge and, along with this, a developing interest in things outside herself. Her previously impaired concept development had made it difficult for her to think in the abstract, resulting in an inability to ask questions about ideas. For the first time she was asking not only "What is colour?", but "Why were the Japanese so strict (meaning cruel) with their prisoners?"

Rikki's steady gains had been exciting because the challenge all along had been a continual problem-solving exercise that was punctuated by small successes, like getting a piece in a puzzle. Each success seemed to lead to one more challenge. Furthermore, Rikki's unfailing optimism, her refusal to give up, her trust in me, all combined to make it impossible for me to give up.

The Agency for the Blind was still unable to supply books on tape, or a cassette player, which was necessary because, at that time, "Talking Books" were incompatible with other systems and could not be played on a regular player. I even approached several publishers to suggest that they might think about producing books on tape, but I was told that I had "a tiger by the tail", and that it would conflict with copyright laws. Then a church committee in the city heard about Rikki and offered to help me with the cost of the tapes. I did not want to re-use them because she liked to listen to them over and over again.

At first the messages from Rikki were repetitive, full of platitudes and failed to give me much feedback about the stories, but she never intentionally criticized anyone in her messages. As her letters increased in length and her ability to express herself improved, the problems she was facing in the institution became more apparent between the lines, and finally became a very real cry for help. The following selections of letters are transcribed from the tapes exactly as spoken by Rikki. They speak so well for themselves that further comment is unnecessary.

MESSAGE NUMBER 1
Wednesday, November 22

The weather is fine. My teacher, Margaret, bought me this tape. How are you? I listened to your tape in the schoolroom. We have a special school here that is part of the institution, but really isn't part of it because it is run separate. I was glad to hear that there is a book called a dictionary. I didn't know that. I am really happy to learn so much from a tape. I listened to it three times.

May I ask you a favour? I want you to thank all my friends at Rehab. I feel I am really neglecting them. I haven't seen them for so long... well... for about ten days. My teacher read me a story about squirrels. I didn't know about squirrels getting into mischief.

I went to Art this week. I did some colouring with my left hand. The teacher said it was good. I am doing very well and I'm working hard and doing my exercises. Today we went cooking and we had that stuff called "Coffee Mate."

I think of you when I go to bed. Here's a joke Sally. What did the stamp say to the letter? It said "I know when I'm licked". Please send another tape soon. I'm watching every day for the mail.

MESSAGE NUMBER 2
Monday, January 15

I went home for Christmas. I got some flowers and a record and we had chip dip. Did I tell you about Chrissie? He is blind too. He's on another ward but I see him at the school. He plays the mouth organ, and can he ever play! What does everyone do on a ski trip? I'm twenty now, so I guess I can do things for myself. I wish I could see you. Chrissie had a party on his birthday. All the people born this week got a cup-cake. How can I learn to fold paper?

Did you hear anything more about getting me a Talking Book machine? Why don't they ever have one? I can cross my right leg right over my left one now. I am always wishing you were here. Someone is teaching me about "take-away" and "borrowing". I will have to put my mind to it. People in the city don't know enough or they would send me that Talking Book machine.

Sometimes I feel kind of bad, but I feel good when your tape comes. It's noisy in the ward, and I can't get the tape recorder because it is locked up, but I can use it in the school room. Here's a joke about coffee. You'll be too old and weak yourself sometime.

MESSAGE NUMBER 3
Thursday, February 1

It's a very good book. It's the best book anyone wrote. I like so much to hear about the bees and the honey and all those things I never knew before. I like the chapter about the wall and that thing called a scorpion. I never saw a toad. But would you do me a favour Sally? What exactly IS a toad?

I went to a church service. I could not go home for the long week-end. I can't tell you the reason, but.... something bad happened in my family. (Prompting in the background.) Well, it was my Grandmother. She died. I couldn't go to the church and now I will never see my Grandmother again. I heard that there are many "nominations", and every one is good.

That's Chrissie, Sally. He plays the mouth-organ. It's really amazing what books you can read because these things we didn't know before and now we do. I just got another cassette in the mail and I can hardly wait to hear it. Today a man came to see me from the government. He asked me how much money I had in the bank. How would I have any money in the bank? But he was nice, and he had a funny accent.

There's a new girl on our ward. Her name is Donna. Sometimes she is lonely and cries, so I am helping her. She is always asking, "Where is Rikki?"

Did anything happen about my eye test? I guess they forgot about it. They're not very smart in the City.

MESSAGE NUMBER 4
Wednesday, February 21

It was kind of hectic the last time I went home. My Mother does all the work, and I really try, because I am too heavy for her. I wish I could walk so I could help.

I think this whole idea of taping every word is working tremendously. It's not just that I get a kick out of it. It's that it gets me in suspense, and I have to wait for the next tape. You asked me to tell you about the story. Well, it's really the best story, and that's the best I can do.

Were you talking to the hospital about my eye test? Please tell me more about that house that you are all trying to get in the City. I really want to go there, and the sooner the better. Why does it take so long to get a house? I guess it is a very hard thing to do, but I just know it is going well, and then I will come and live there.

Do you ever see Dan? It makes me think about when you and Dan put me on a horse. Lord knows when that will ever happen again. If you see Dan, tell me, because I am quite excited. Yesterday Lally's back was very sore. She can't talk much, but the staff helps her. She writes poetry. She had a weak spell. If we can cheer her up, we have to.

If you could send me some blank tapes it would be good, just some without anything on, so I can write to you, and please send me the next part of the story.

MESSAGE NUMBER 5
Monday, March 5

I nearly died when I read about those dogs called Widdle and Puke, and the shaggy dog called Dodo! I love everything we've been doing so much I just started to cry. These stories are really interesting. It's a very good book.

Nobody ever told me about these things. Nobody ever talks about things like that here.

I was shocked when you told me you were resigning. I guess it's important if you have to go to school again, but that's funny, because I thought you knew everything. Here, you don't go to school after you are twenty-one, so how can *you* go to school?

But I'm wondering when you are going to resign, because it's a sad thing to hear, and I don't know what to say. I can't really express it. Will you still be able to send me some tapes? And one more thing, Sally, what does "shaggy" mean?

Now I am going to ask you a question. That man came back from the government. He asked me if I could sign my name and I said "No Sir", but I had to mark six papers that had my name on them. I don't know what they said, but he was asking all those questions again about how much money I had in the bank. He said he was from South America - just crazy - talking away, and talking away. I told him I had never been in a bank. He spoke funny. I told him I always put my mind into what I did and he said he would come again.

Why are people from the city so strange? I told him if I didn't have you I wouldn't be doing these things and he said he hadn't met you, so I guess you don't know who he is. He said he was going to try to help me, but I don't know what he would do. Do you think he would get me into that house?

MESSAGE NUMBER 6

Monday, March 19

This taping is incredible! Now I can get the tape in and out myself fast. I didn't know animals would do these things. I am really amazed. In your tape you asked me again to tell you about what I thought. Well - books are hard to choose - what to do - after we get to the next book I'll give you my opinion of it. These books are really good, and I am beginning to realize that.

I'm trying to get Lally to talk on tape, but she's afraid. She has a very soft voice. Sometimes you think she hasn't any voice at all. Next week I can't send a tape because it will be school break here, and the machine isn't allowed on the ward. It would get smashed. Today I played Bingo and I bounced a ball. We had some water and we found out what floats. I was amazed. A lot of things surprise me and that was one of them.

May I ask you a stupid question. That man who came - Lally said he was black. His skin was all black, instead of white. Are people different colours? That is - I guess God made everything black and white - like night and day, or like chocolate cake and white cake, so I guess that's why. But does it make any real difference if someone is black or some other colour instead of white? How do people get black?... Sometime, would you tell me about colour - I mean ... not in people ... just colour, like green, and yellow, and brown. What is it really like? I'd like to know about that.

Well, down every road there's a city. At least that's what they say.

MESSAGE NUMBER 7
Tuesday, April 3

It's not easy. It's really a difficult task. I really have to concentrate to answer the questions. I asked my teacher if she would put on a tape with questions on it so I could practice. I never answered questions before, so my mind has to learn how to do it.

I was talking to my supervisor about getting "Talking Books". My teacher wrote a letter. I told her we had asked them a million times, and guess what - they sent a book back in Braille! I never could read that much Braille, and anyway, I can't feel it. What I need is tapes that I can put on and listen to. But I guess I'll never get them. These people in the City never understand.

In the winter I can't even get outside and when it rains the program is canceled, so I can hardly wait to go to Camp. Then I can get outside, and there is water, and swimming. They help you. It's right on a big river and it's fantastic. If you saw it you would like it. If you would like to go maybe I could arrange it. I had to *really* concentrate on the questions. I had to *really* study. My teacher sent those books back... Just a minute... It's a quarter after two by my clock. I always know the time now.

Camp Open House is in July. I know you are busy, but could you come?

MESSAGE NUMBER 8

Monday, June 4

Is there anything I can do for you? Everything is going well here. I like this ward much better except that there is hardly anyone I can talk to except the staff, and they are always too busy.

Sometimes I talk to Chrissie and Lally and I tell them about the stories. Lally wants to know if you could send her some stories too. I don't want to let her have my tapes because they would get lost or broken.

What would it be like to go to another country? I would like to show your friends what I can do, but they are all very, very smart. They should go to Switzerland. How do people learn English?

Excuse me. I have to check my clock. If I didn't have this clock I don't know what I would do. That last tape sort of gave me a boost in an idea. You said there were many other kinds of stories. This story - I just laughed and laughed. But you said... not mystery... no, not mystery... it was biography. That was the word. You said we would do a variety. But I am going well on it and these last stamps are my last, so can you send me some more?

You said you were going to see a lady in the public library to see if they will put books on tape. She will probably think you are crazy, but all we want is for people to hear them, because the Agency hasn't got them, and then maybe some other people will want them too. Maybe a hundred, or even a thousand.

I had a crazy dream last night. I thought you were "barking me out", and you said "*listen!*" and I woke up and started crying and crying. I don't think this ever happened to me before - like thinking something was happening in my sleep when I wasn't even awake. Could you please come to Open House? I need to see you.

MESSAGE NUMBER 9
Monday, June 11

I feel guilty, not speaking French. Maybe if I learned a word at a time I could. Today I saw a tulip. And there is this Patricia Hearst on the news. She's gone "bonkers" -- that's what they say now. It's a horrible feeling inside for parents to say, that is my daughter, and look at her now.

Thank you for sending the first test about the story. I want to tell you something. I'm doing things now I've never done before, and that's about these questions. You ask me to say "yes" or "no", and sometimes I can do things I never knew I could do.

Can you come to "Open House"? I hope so. If you want to know a question, tell me, just leave a space, and I can tell you the answer. There's no reason why all these questions cannot be ironed out, so just fire away. At least that's what I think anyway.

Maybe it's none of my business, but I'd like to know something. When is your birthday? I want to get you something. Everyone is always helping me. Now I want to help someone. I do my exercises every day, push-ups and all that stuff. Woodwork was cancelled to-day. It's lucky I've got this clock. When one of the staff didn't have a watch I said, "I can tell you what time it is," and I did. They were surprised. I'm just too good-hearted. I can tell time real good now. But it took you and me a long time to find out how a clock works. As you said, I should put my hands away back on my wheelchair when I am moving somewhere. If you don't, you don't know where you are. There aren't any grab bars here so I can't get on the toilet, but you could tell them how. Please excuse all the noise on this tape, but Chrissie and Harry are here.

I am enjoying every bit of the story, so please send the next, and I am out of stamps.

MESSAGE NUMBER 10
Monday, June 16

I got a tape in the mail yesterday. You said the story was on side B and the explaining was on side A. That's a good thing - the explaining, that is, because now I know what I didn't know before, about the questions, I mean, and what the right answer is. It really gives me the idea of how you do these things that I never knew before.

The times that I can listen to the stories, well, this is a difficult thing because, as you know, I will have to try to listen in the ward office because soon it will be the holidays. The ward is so noisy sometimes I can hardly hear anything.

I don't know what got me going so well about this clock, but suddenly I knew about the "before" and "after" and I could tell the time. I'm thinking that I could learn to tell money too if I had a chance. But the Tuck Shop is upstairs and no one in wheelchairs can go. Sometimes Chrissie goes up. You can get a chocolate bar or a cup of coffee there if you have some money. They cost quite a lot.

We were given by a church group a box of clothes and also some cookies. I don't need any clothes, because my family gets them for me, but sometimes my Mum gets cross if someone else wears my things. Again I'm putting my hopes too high, but I hope they are getting that house soon. I just know they are, because they are all very smart, and they don't give up.

I really think I've got a good thing with these tapes. I promise I will keep going. I won't quit. It is not easy to concentrate when there are thirty kids around, and all of them making a racket. There are some spots I miss, but I just play the tape again and then I understand.

They keep sending me those big Braille books. We told them not to send them, but they just keep coming every week.

MESSAGE NUMBER 11
Monday, July 23

I'm glad you came to see me at Camp. Now you know what it's like. I think it's fantastic. I had a good time. Someone sent some tapes but they don't sound good, and one got caught in the machine so we couldn't use it for a long time. It had to go to "Maintenance".

It's hard to find a place to work now because it's holidays. We have a teacher here for the summer named Tammy. At least I think she's a teacher. She's giving me lessons on a chord organ.

I got the questions about "My Family and Other Animals". They are quite hard. I have to play the tape over and over to get the answer. I'm going to miss Gerald Durrell. I sort of got to know him, and now we are starting something different. It's a very good story, don't get me wrong, I like it a lot, but I got used to the other one, and now we have something that is not the same, and the name is "Just So Stories". I really liked the one about the cat. I never saw a cat but I think they are soft. One thing I would like to know is what is "best beloved"?

I got the stamps and Tammy helped me put them on all the envelopes so they won't get lost. It really shocks me to know all these things I didn't know before - like stamps on letters - and now I do. Please send me another tape soon.

MESSAGE NUMBER 12
Thursday, August 20

Here is a tune on the organ. My teacher is a volunteer. The trouble is, the organ has to be locked up so that it won't get damaged, and I can't practice. But I'm allowed to have my radio during the day now if I keep it on my lap all the time. I listen to music and the news.

Could I ask you a question? With horses, there are colts, and they are the boy horses, and fillies, and they are the girl horses, but if they don't talk, then what really is the difference? Also could you please tell me what "inflation" is?

My teacher is telling me about tone and volume, but I don't quite get it - the difference, that is. But if at first you don't succeed, try, try again. That's my motto.

I've gotten over being sensitive. I'm just too kind-hearted and sensitive. I just know everything will work out. I will do anything to help. I will not let you down. You know, and I know too, that you can't count your chickens before they're hatched....

MESSAGE NUMBER 13
Thursday, September 20

I'm sorry I was so long with this tape, but I was busy - well, that is, it was hard to get it set up on the ward and the staff are very busy these days. Today it's bad news because now I am twenty-one, and I can't go to school any more. That's the cut-off. It is the rule.

But sometimes I don't understand. My counselor says, if I am so smart, how come I can't tie my shoe laces? There is a place here called Community Skills. It is run by Marianne. She says that I have to tie my shoe laces and make my bed if I want to pass Community Skills. Right now my counselor is teaching me my colours. We have one shape that is red and one that is blue and so on.

If I didn't have this tape recorder I don't know what I would do. I can't seem to get hold of a social worker out here, but I want to know more about that house. I just know they are going to get it and then I will move out. I don't care what it's like, I will like it. What do people do at the university?

MESSAGE NUMBER 14
Tuesday, October 9

I am a nervous wreck, trying to answer those questions. Is my "contrast" getting better? What you said about how people talk - loud and soft and that - but you said mistakes don't matter, because that's how we learn - by mistakes, even if you have to go "on punishment" sometimes - that's how you learn.

I am also glad because you don't give up on me and you don't give up on that house. You are not a quitter, and I am not a quitter, and that makes two of us. You said you are busy right now. How do you find time to make these tapes? And you have to write essays. What actually are essays? Could you send me one?

My machine was locked up but I have it to-day. I'm in the back room where it is not too noisy right now. Why do horses have shoes on in summer and take them off in winter, that's what I'd like to know. That may be a silly question, but you said no questions are silly, because when you don't know, that's how you find out.

Australia is a hot place. That's what the story said. I guess thirst really "quenches" in hot places. Everything will work out. Don't get me wrong. I'm really working at these questions. Now this Legacy, I know what that is, and about Australia, and how the whole world is round like a round ball. No one ever told me these things, and now I know.

I think Nevil Shute is a good writer. He is the best I have read. And now I know that when it is night in Australia it is day here. About those Japanese. I don't know how they could be so "strict" with the prisoners - that's what I can't understand.

You said that you phoned the Agency and they never called back. Well, that's just what they are like, and if they don't help people, how can people manage?

Do you think I could get a job off the ward? I am doing some tests with the Community Skills Department to see if I can move out of here. That's a good thing, but some of these things are very hard, like telling dark clothes from light clothes for the wash. How can I do that?

MESSAGE NUMBER 15

Monday, November 12

I'm feeling kind of low to-day. The Community Skills Program turned me down. They said I couldn't do any Community Skills - things like preparing a meal, making my bed, tying my shoe laces, washing my hair. Some of those things in the kitchen, like a "flower sifter" - why do people sift flowers anyway?

It's not like the Rehab we had in the City at all. You said I did well in that Rehab. Do you think if you talked to them they would change their mind? What tests do I have to pass to get into that house?

When they told me I just cried and cried. If you spoke to them they would listen, but my counselor says I am just too big for my shoes.

I really miss all my friends in the city. I feel guilty about them. Maybe I should pay them a visit. I need to practice some of those things again, like transfers to the bath and toilet because here I can't do those things. They don't even have a bath here. They just put you on the slab and hose you down - and if the water is too cold, well, too bad.

Don't get me wrong. The staff here are very good to me. I can't really explain it. It's just that when I was there all the staff found that there were lots of things I could do, and here they don't want you to do any of those things. The staff are always busy because there are so many people here who can't do anything. And there is no quiet place, not anywhere. Sometimes I see Chrissie. He wants to go to that house too.

Please send another tape soon because I want to know what happens to those people in Malaya.

MESSAGE NUMBER 16
Monday, December 12

Hello Sally. This is Rikki. Today it is December the twelfth and it is almost Christmas. My Dad will come and get me. That really shocks me, how you are getting that home, and how long it takes to fill out all the forms for the government, getting By-Laws and Corporations and all that. I never knew about all those things, and how long it takes. All those people must be very smart. Please let me know if I can help.

Sally, may I ask a question, and you can say no if you like. When I go home for Christmas, could I see you? I know you are very busy and you have your family, but if I could just see you for a short time I would feel good. If the answer is no I will understand. I'm so good-hearted, I wish I could do something for you. What would you like for Christmas? You just name it and I will get it.

I was reading the story of the "Incredible Journey" again. This story really gets me. Those animals are really smart, smarter than some people I think. The people went and left them and they found their way and didn't even get lost. I think that is really smart. But one thing I don't know -- what is a mine?

Please send the next tape soon. I don't know what I would do without these stories. I'm going to take my entire tapes home with me for Christmas and listen to them all again.

MESSAGE NUMBER 17

Sunday, January 8

I am still singing all that music I heard at the concert. Just seeing you was one thing, but going to a real concert was something I never thought I would do that and I still can't believe that the sound was so beautiful. I have never heard a whole orchestra before and now I just love ballet music.

And now I know what a theatre is like, with all the seats in rows, with some in front and some behind. I never knew that before. You are working so hard at the university and with those people about the house. I don't know how you will have time, but I hope you will not stop sending me the tapes. When I was home I listened to all my tapes for eleven hours. My Dad said I would have a sore bum or a sore ear -- one or the other, but I used my headphones. I never get tired of listening to these tapes.

What is that music you put on tape? It is another big orchestra like the Nutcracker, and it is a really good tune. But I have to use my head-phones, because the staff say they don't like that kind of music. They say it is "classical". What does that mean?

I was shocked at all the questions you sent on side B. I didn't know there could be so many questions. How could you think them all up? I had to play the tape over and over to fill in all the blanks, and some might be wrong because some things I don't understand. But you said to fill it in with whatever I thought, and if it is wrong, you will send me the right answer, and then I will learn. We really have a good idea here, for example, I am not sure how much money it will cost Jean to buy a well full of drinking water but I guess it would cost a lot.

You asked if I would like to read another book by Gerald Durrell. Yes I would because I really miss that family. That's how it is with books.

MESSAGE NUMBER 18
Monday, February 13

You get to know them, and then they are gone, and you miss them. I would like to hear more about them. But you said it is good to get used to other writers too. Maybe we could read another by Nevil Shute, because he is such a good writer, at least that's what I think.

Now, that story about the boy called Tom Sawyer, that's different. I just don't seem to get on to it. It's not that I don't like it. It was the same with the "Book of Small", about that artist. It was hard to keep on with, if you know what I mean. I hope you won't mind if I say that, but the other books are better.

One thing I want to tell you, Sally. Someone came to see me from that house you are getting in the city. They asked me a lot of questions about why I wanted to go and all that, and I had to mark an "X" on the paper. Do you know who they were? Are they getting the house soon? They said they couldn't tell me anything yet, until the committee meets again, but now I am really curious. I know you'll let me know about it.

MESSAGE NUMBER 19
Monday, March 13

Today I am not feeling very well. I guess I am heart-sick. I cried all night last night because I got a letter. I guess you know. That committee turned me down for the house. They said I had to be more independent. But how can I, when I can't even try things out? I just know I could, if they would only give me a chance. Community Skills told them I couldn't pass the test. Can you say something to them? They would listen to you. They just don't know all the things I can do now that I never knew before.

It's hard to do questions because of the ward and there is no quiet room. You can hear it on the tape. They are always shouting and hollering and all that, and sometimes my room-mate has screaming fits. She just screams and screams. I am in the small room off the ward with Peggy, Alice and Julie, and I have a small table, but if Peggy is "on punishment" then all the rest of us have to get out.

Chrissie is going to be moved from his ward to a new ward. They are starting a new plan for the blind and Chrissie was picked. That's all I know.

MESSAGE NUMBER 20
Monday, March 20

I've been watching the mail every day for your reply to my last message, and today it came. I've been crying ever since I got that letter about the house, and now I am crying again from happiness after getting your tape, because you said that you are coming here, not just to visit, but actually on staff. Now I know that I'm going to get out of here some day, and that you won't give up on me.

Will you still be able to read to me when you come? You said that you will be working as a leader on the new ward for the blind. They won't let me go to that ward because they don't want any wheelchairs on it. Will you be able to work with me too?

Chrissie is going on that ward, and his friends Harry and Peer and Rory. I don't know how they got picked, but I guess they are all blind and they can all walk. Sometimes Peer gets really mad and he has to go "on punishment". He punches people out when he is angry.

I hope you come soon. I'm counting the time on my clock. It makes me feel good when I think of it. And now you will teach me more and more things and I will get into that house. There's one thing about us, Sally. We never quit.

PART 3 - THE INSTITUTION

Chapter 9

PLANS AND EXPECTATIONS

"You can never plan the future by the past."
Edmund Burke

The institution was set back and up from the highway, so that only the skyline was visible from the road. As you approached, it gradually grew taller on the horizon until it looked like a small town, with the Canadian flag fluttering in the wind at the south end, and the power house chimneys belching smoke at the other.

The long entrance driveway forked at the top of the hill to form a perimeter road that encircled the entire complex. Parking areas with neat rows of cars nestled into the lee of the wings, like a child's model village.

Spacious grounds surrounded the building as far as the horizon in all directions, like a well-kept, but deserted, golf course. September colours were beginning to show in the trees and shrubs, but the well-tended flower beds of yellow chrysanthemums and red geraniums were still untouched by frost.

Looking down from above, the buildings might have looked like a giant shopping plaza, with six wings crossing the main artery that was over a mile in length.

Standing at the north end, and looking down the long corridor was like looking through a giant telescope with a light at the far end, but looking from the south end there was no light so that the corridor seemed to go on to infinity.

My first impression was that it could house the entire town, and I may have been nearly right because this was one of the town's main sources of employment. Many such institutions were built in Canada around the same time, in the 1920s, all with a similar architectural plan, to provide residential care for the mentally retarded population.

People used to say that all government facilities for the retarded were built in remote areas so that they would be "out of sight and out of mind". This was partly true, because at that time, people who are now called developmentally delayed or mentally challenged were not considered capable of learning or of making any contribution to society. Parents were advised to institutionalize such children who would otherwise place intolerable stress upon the family, because at that time there was no form of community support.

Even today, although the government provides partial Home Care and education, the cost in time, strength, and finances becomes intolerable, particularly for the mother in the family. Younger children in the family are affected, and when the disabled child grows older, the health and strength of the parents declines too. Eventually some form of placement may be required.

Maplegrove Center For The Mentally Retarded was situated on the outskirts of the small town of Burnside. Many of the large government institutions, like Maplegrove, were constructed in the 1920"s and located in economically depressed areas of the country in order to boost employment. This was an articulated government objective. Some were located in regions that had lost the main town employer due to modernization or re-location of the industry. At that time, in the 1920s, Maplegrove had a capacity for 2500 residents. Now there were 1600 and about the same number of staff.

My first day at Maplegrove consisted of the usual orientation to a new job, signing the contract, meeting with the staff, having the required health tests and general orientation.

On the second day I attended my first meeting with the Resource Team for the new ward for blind residents. This "pilot project" was initiated by the government, initially to determine the number of residents who had serious vision problems, and then to select suitable candidates for a special ward, where training programs to meet their special needs could be carried out.

The meeting was to be held in an empty ward that had been designated as the new location for the program. As I entered the room I was reminded of a huge warehouse. It was sparsely furnished for the meeting, with a few ill-matching chairs and tables set against one pale green wall in need of a coat of paint. The room smelled stale. As team members approached their footsteps echoed and their voices sounded hollow in the empty room. Chairs were dragged unwillingly over to form a semi-circle for the conference.

Stanley Binks, the unit director, had called the meeting to plan the procedure for implementing the project. I had met so many new people the previous day that I despaired of ever remembering all their names. Stanley introduced me to the first three counselors to join the team, Howard Sylvester, Ron King and Darlene Kenny, as well as Philip Martin, the social worker who had attended the case conference at Rehab. Dr. Peter Ambrose, the medical director, had not yet arrived.

"Good party at the Legion last night," observed Ron. "What time did you get home, Stan?"

"None of your business, Ron," laughed Stanley. Some playful bantering followed while everyone arranged seats and secured paper and pen.

"How much help can we expect from the Government on this, Stan?" asked Howard. "There's quite a bit of discontent about it on the other wards. They think the staff ratio is unfair. How do we handle that?"

"That's what this meeting's all about, Howard," said Stanley. "You all know why we're here -- to open a ward for blind or very low vision residents and provide specialized training for future community living. This is not just custodial care. It's something new. We've got Sally here now to help us with the program. The wards have all submitted their lists of residents who might benefit the most and we're ready to get started. You three got some training at the Agency for the Blind. You're going to have a chance to put that knowledge to the test now, and we want your suggestions. First, we have to set up priorities. What we do first, how we do it, who does it -- that kind of thing. Where do you come in Sally? Perhaps you could tell us now what your role's going to be."

"Thank you Stanley," I replied. "First I'd like to say that I'm pleased to be working with all of you. I realize that we all have different skills and backgrounds, so we're each going to contribute something different. My role, as an occupational therapist, will be to help with assessments, leading to developing training programs. Essentially, that means that we want to assure that each resident understands what he's being taught, and that it's presented at the right level for him. And we'll need some specialized equipment and furnishings. I understand that until now, the blind residents have been scattered throughout the entire institution, on wards with sighted residents, and we're going to be able to change that. Each one of you has had experience going blindfolded onto a ward. What did you learn from that?"

There was silence for a moment. Then Darlene said, "I was scared. I never knew what was coming at me. It's not just the problem of bumping into something, but when someone comes and grabs you, or tries to guide you by taking your arm or steering you by the neck or shoulder when you can't see... Well, it was all I could do not to rip off the blindfold. I can understand now why you're supposed to let a blind person take *your* arm."

"What about you, Ron," I asked.

"Oh, I don't know," said Ron. "I guess I was using my ears more... Like hearing the sound of the room so I could tell where I was. But it was so noisy. I kept bumping into things - or people."

"I did too," said Howard. "I felt like a boxer. Remember poor old Poddy, who always had a banged-up nose? I just kept my arms out in front, but that doesn't help you with low objects, and the edge of the door is the "shits"."

"You've all raised some good points," I said. "I think my biggest problem was not knowing how the sighted residents would react when I walked into them, if they didn't understand that I couldn't see, but also the noise level. So now we'll understand the need to arrange the furniture in a certain way, and not change it. We also have to keep the noise level down so the residents can make better use of their hearing. Let's look at the list of residents who seem to have the most potential for this new ward. Am I right in saying that all of them can walk independently, we're not taking anyone in a wheelchair, and they all have good hearing, good balance, and some learning ability?"

"Yes," said Ron. "They have an average age of twenty-one. One is fourteen, and one is thirty, but they're mostly in their teens or early twenties. You all know that the purpose of this program is to provide special needs training for blind residents. By this we mean that there will be a kind of special teaching approach, to try to teach them to help themselves a bit, find their way around and maybe even learn some work skills. We don't know yet how much we're going to be able to teach them, but they've been selected because none of them have any severe behavior problems and they're all able to walk. This is a very different approach from the other wards."

"And with only eighteen instead of thirty we should be able to give a lot more individual attention," said Darlene.

"Remember Jackie, on Ward D?" asked Ron. "He was never allowed to walk because the staff were afraid he'd get hurt, not being able to see where he was going."

"Good point, Ron," I said, "and that was probably because the ward was so noisy and crowded that you or I would have had the same problem if we couldn't see. How is the girls' washroom coming along, Ron?"

"The door's on order, Sally. Should come any day now," replied Ron. "Then it's going to be up to you guys to teach the boys not to go into the girls'."

"Do you think we're going to have any problems with this co-ed arrangement, Stanley?" asked Howard.

"It's the Government's idea, not ours," replied Stanley. "Never been done before. Some parents refused consent for this reason. I guess that's something we're just going to have to find out."

"Most of the guys don't even know there's a sex difference," said Howard. "That's just one thing they're going to learn too, up to a point. How do we teach sexuality to a blind person? You can't very well allow them to feel everyone, can you?" Everyone laughed.

"They'd just better not find out for a while," laughed Howard. "Let's not invite problems. We'll have enough as it is."

"OK," said Stanley. "Let's write out the strategy so far. The whole ward has to be painted. Then we bring in the furniture, the female cots go into the sunrooms, three in each, and the washroom is cut in half. Then we start phasing in, twelve male, six female. Darlene, you haven't said anything. Do you have any questions?"

Darlene thought for a moment. "I just don't see how it's all going to work, Stanley. How are we going to know what to do? Gee, with all of them blind, I don't know. Where do we start? How many will we have at once? The course at the Agency for the Blind gave us some idea of how to work with them, but they weren't talking about people who were so disabled. I just don't know how what we learned is going to apply to these guys."

"Good grief, Darlene!" exclaimed Stanley. "Don't get cold feet at this point! You volunteered to come on this ward."

"May I say something?" said Philip, a Social Worker, who had remained silent until now. "As I understand it, Stanley, we're going to phase in a few at a time. We start with the highest functioning, like Chrissie and Peer, then bring in one or two a day as we can handle them. There's no need to panic. Nobody's saying that they all have to come at once, and there's no time limit. Do you agree with that Sally?"

"Yes, of course, Philip. But it's particularly important to take Chrissie, Harry and Rory together. They've been together most of their lives and it would be a big mistake to separate them now, even for a short time.

"I once read about two women," I continued, "both with severe cerebral palsy and comprehending everything but unable to talk normally. Their beds were side-by-side. They quickly recognized each other's intellectual abilities and, together, they developed and learned an intricate system of communication. They became close companions, although no one was aware of this. One day one of them was put into a wheelchair and moved to another ward. Later she was able to learn to communicate through Bliss Symbolics, and it was then that she was able to explain how traumatic this separation from her friend had been for both of them.

"Communication is going to be a big factor in our program, and we have to recognize the importance of relationships among our residents, and not destroy their friendships. We're all going to have to communicate a great deal, and start at a very basic level, along with basic self-care skills, mobility and orientation. We'll have to get some carpeting in right away for down the centre of the ward, to help them find their way."

"Carpeting, Sally?" asked Ron. "My Gosh, this is still an institution you know, not a private club."

"Change your thinking, Ron," I said. "Our job is to see that these residents have everything they need to learn. Their environment is going to be very important. One way blind people can find their way around is by changes in floor surface."

"Does that go for equipment too?" asked Darlene. "Can we get our own sports equipment, Braille watches, and things like that?"

"Gee, I don't know, Darlene," said Ron. "We haven't even been given a budget yet. What do you say, Sally?"

"As I understand it, Ron, we make up the budget. But we have to do it in the proper order and not rush out and get the wrong things. Braille watches may be a little ahead of the game. We'd better look at tooth brushes first. But I think we can get anything that's justified."

"Then I'd say let's go for it," said Howard. "And let's move fast before the Government changes its mind. There could be a new minister next year and the whole thing could be scrapped."

"I'm not that pessimistic," I said. "We can make up a list of basics today to send in and you can all add to it. Can the beds be moved in tomorrow, right after the painting?"

"That's the plan," said Stanley. "Beds tomorrow, linen Tuesday, everything else within the next two or three weeks."

"Do we get a chesterfield and some easy chairs?" asked Darlene. "We can make this half of the ward into a living room. We'll need some shelves, and tables too."

"Now you're thinking more positive," said Howard, "What do you think about having some exercise mats Sally?"

"Sure, Howard, but now we're getting on to programming, and maybe Philip doesn't want to sit in on that."

"True, Sally," said Philip, "but I thought Dr. Ambrose was coming to this meeting. Will someone be seeing him? We can hardly make decisions without him."

"Oh, he'll go along with anything," said Stanley. "He doesn't like meetings - won't sign his name to anything anyway. He's only too happy to see us doing the work."

"Let's all meet again tomorrow to plan the phasing in," I said.

"Not me," said Howard. "That's my day off."

"Now, just a minute," I said, indignantly. "Stanley, that's something that has to be changed. Howard is essential to this program. We all are. This shift business has to be worked out to free this team to work the same hours for the next few weeks."

"Well, I don't know, Sally," said Stanley. "That's hard to change. I think you'll have to manage without Howard if it's his day off."

"Stanley, this is a new venture. The old ways have to be changed. We need all of us working the same shift, not evenings or weekends, until this ward is humming. We'll have to have meetings every day. All the members of this team must be full time day shift people. We can use part time staff to take over night shift and irregular hours. Communication is going to be the most important thing."

Stanley said he would look into it.

I walked with Philip as far as the stairs. "I'm glad you're here, Sally," he said. "You're like a breath of fresh air. This is the most exciting thing that's happened here in twenty-five years. I'm amazed that the Government had the imagination to do it."

"There must have been a reason, Philip. What do you think happened?"

"I think it was probably that report by that professor of sociology about blind Canadians, Philip. "It was actually commissioned by the Agency for the Blind, but it was a seething attack on both the Government and the agencies for the blind, particularly Government institutions like this, where blind people have been hidden away for years without any special services. Why did you come, Sally?"

"For the same reason, in a way, Philip. I learned about this institution from a patient who was assigned to me at Rehab. She's spent over ten years of her life here, except for a short period at Rehab., and really isn't retarded, although she's grown up to think she is. At Rehab., after only a few weeks, many of us were certain that she wasn't retarded. I just couldn't see how this could happen."

"Yes, I remember that case. It was Rikki Chase. But why did she come back if she wasn't retarded?"

"Good question, Philip. She shouldn't have. But she had no alternative. I came because I was curious to find out how many more there might be like her. Perhaps if there were enough, something might be done. I heard that the Government wanted a resource person to help with this ward, and that there are over a hundred blind residents here. That's quite a lot."

"Yes, and there are quite a lot of deaf here too. I wonder how they were tested. I thought they all had to be certified retarded in order to be admitted."

"Of course they were, Philip. But that's another reason why I came. Do you know what tests were used for these people? They were designed entirely for sighted people. How can you answer a question that depends on vision if you're blind? How can you answer at all if you don't understand language, or if you haven't had the necessary experience to answer the question. Take, for example, a word association question like "nail". When Rikki answered "finger" it was marked wrong. The correct answer was "hammer", but Rikki had never seen or felt a hammer. That's a test of her experience, not her intelligence. Experience and intelligence are linked, but they're not the same thing."

"I see what you mean, Sally. That's terrible, isn't it? Well, I'm glad you're here. We needed someone from outside to get this thing going." Philip opened the door to the stairway. "But don't let them get you down. It won't be easy, you know. The staff aren't used to change around here. Don't try to go too fast. You're coming in from outside, and outsiders don't have a habit of staying."

"I can handle it," I said.

I heard the door shut as I walked down the long corridor that I had already labeled in my mind as "Main Street". Here there were people of all sizes and shapes. I had never before seen so many misshapen people, some with canes or crutches, some in wheelchairs or on stretchers, some standing in the middle of the hallway, or sitting against the wall just watching the world go by.

One resident reached out for me as I walked by. Another began an unintelligible conversation and was still talking to me after I had passed by. Many smiled a greeting, some wanted to hold my hand. One small boy asked if I was his mother. I wondered if he really knew what a mother was, and what to say, except perhaps "I wish I were". I wondered what this question really meant to him. Did that boy have any real concept of "mother", or a vague recollection of his own mother? Or was he just repeating something he had heard others say? Did I give him the right answer? The corridor was busy and noisy, and it was necessary to weave around the floor cleaners, food wagons, maintenance ladders and various types of equipment as well as people.

The staff wore no uniforms or identity labels, and as I progressed down the long hallway it occurred to me that it was not always obvious who were employees and who were residents. I thought about the meeting and the plans for the new ward. I wondered what sort of results we would get. A lot would depend on the resourcefulness and motivation of the staff. None of them had had any previous experience in anything like this, but then, neither had I.

I wondered how the staff had been selected. Had they all volunteered, and if so, why? Were they looking on this as a reprieve from a dull, thankless, repetitive job where no improvement was expected? Did any of them have any idea what rehabilitation was all about, or any real interest in the teaching aspects of the job? Darlene's fears were well founded. I wondered how much ability any of us would have to bring about change in these people who had had so little advantage in the past.

If a person's character is formed by his environment as much as by heredity, if you were to radically alter the environment, surely behavior would be affected. I decided that the only way to approach it would be to do what I had done with Rikki and take each day as it came. I did not realize, at that time, that the results would far exceed anyone's expectations.

Chapter 10

THE IMPOSSIBLE IS ONLY THE UNTRIED

"There is no handicap in blindness. The handicap is in idleness."
Helen Keller

It was three days later when I finally had time to talk to Rikki. Attending meetings, ordering equipment, writing reports and letters, and myriads of paper work in addition to meeting new staff and finding my way around occupied me completely. I discovered that just walking from one end of "Main Street" to the other took half an hour.

Rikki's delight at "seeing" me again caused the usual waterfall of tears of joy. "Now I really know you're going to get me out of here," she cried, wiping the back of her hand across her wet face.

"I'm still on the Planning Committee for the group home," I said, "so we'll just keep working on it. In the meantime, we'll continue with your therapy and see how much more you can learn."

"I wish I could be on that ward."

"Never mind, Rikki. You need a different kind of training. We'll have a program for you too, even if you're not on the special ward."

We were sitting in the sunroom at the back of her ward. Four cots, a white metal table and a straight-backed chair filled the room, with just enough space for her to maneuver with her wheelchair.

"This next bed is Peggy's," Rikki was saying. "She's deaf so she never hears anything and she can't talk. The next bed is Alice. She often screams at night and has to be told to shut up. The last one is Julie. She's just like a baby. She likes to sit for hours and hours in the corner. Sometimes I talk to her, but she never answers. I think she's lonely."

"Is there anyone here you *can* talk to, Rikki?"

"Not really - not like you and me. They're all retarded, you know. They talk, but it doesn't make any sense… like saying the same words over and over. Patsy, over there, is always picking up things and saying "Look at me. Look what I've got." She gets attention that way." Rikki lowered her voice.

"I've got three good friends, though. They're not on this ward, but they're good friends. I see them sometimes, and we talk about getting out of here."

"Are they blind too, Rikki?"

"One is - Chrissie, but not the others. And I'm the only blind one on this ward. Lally has weak spells and has to be in a special wheelchair, and Pinky was born with no arms and legs so she has to have everything done for her. But they are my very best friends, and I love them both."

"Why is it that you can't be together with your friends, Rikki?"

"It's the rule. Once you come into this place, you STAY PUT, PERIOD! You never change wards. That is the rule. And you never change units. This unit is for people over fourteen. Then there is Unit One. It's for people who are like babies. Unit Two is for children, and Unit Three is for people who are real "crackers" - you know - real problems. Thank God I'm not on Unit Three. I'd go clean out of my mind. I'd..."

"Are Lally and Pinky on Unit Three then?"

"Oh no. I'd never see them if they were. They're on this unit, but on a different ward. I see them when I go to Choir, or sometimes in the dining room. Pinky's a good singer. We sing duets sometimes. She wants to be a real singer some day."

"Where do you keep your things, Rikki... your clothes, your radio and tape recorder? Do you have a dresser or cupboard?"

"Oh no, Sally. Everything's locked up in the ward office cupboards. They would get ruined on the ward."

"Are there any books to read? Does anyone read to you?"

"Books aren't allowed on the wards. All the books are kept in the school, and that is the Board of Education. And I can't go there any more because I'm twenty-one. No one is ever allowed to talk to the teachers. They are out of bounds, except for one day every year. That is the "Meet the Teachers" day. And they're not allowed to come here. The wards and the school are completely separate."

"Are you sure of that Rikki? I don't understand why we would not be able to talk to the teachers. How would the staff know what's going on?"

"You'll find out Sally. You won't be able to talk to them either, now that you're on staff."

"Who goes to school, Rikki? Why aren't you going when you were doing so well ?"

"I was allowed to go for a short time when I came back from Rehab., because they asked, but as soon as I turned twenty-one, no more school. That's the cut-off age. Mrs. Jones helped me a lot, but she isn't really a teacher for the blind. It's mostly small children who go. I don't know what they do there, but they must do something, because quite a lot go. Well Sally, the way I look at it is this. I want to get on with it, so I'll do anything. But here? Well, I guess I'm too old for this school."

"Would you like to go to a real school if you had a chance? You see, Rikki, no one is ever really too old for school. I go to school sometimes. Lots of adults go to school, but under different programs than this. Maybe we could start our own school program just for you. We'll have to find a quiet place to work, and a place where we can leave the equipment out for you to use."

Rikki lowered her voice. "Pardon me, Sally, but you're new here. I don't think that will be possible here."

"Nothing is impossible, Rikki."

Suddenly the shrill voice of a counselor called out, "Everyone line up for dinner!"

Several women had been standing in a line in the hallway for almost an hour, large white bibs tied around their necks. Slowly others began to join them, and the line began to move down the corridor towards the dining room. I decided to follow and see how Rikki managed at the table.

The dining room reminded me of Dickens' "Oliver Twist". Over a hundred residents from all the wards on the Unit were seated at long tables amid a din of loud voices mingled with the clatter of dishes and scraping of chairs along the floor. Kitchen staff hurried around, placing dinner plates of food, a glass of milk, and a slice of bread at each place. Few needed any urging to dig in, eating as best they could, many encircling their food with their arms and stuffing as much as they could into their mouths at once. Few bothered with utensils. Table manners were unknown, the business of eating was all that mattered, but sometimes more food seemed to be destined for faces, hands and floor than for the mouth.

Some residents on all wards needed to be fed by the staff, and they were kept back on the wards. This procedure required staff with extraordinary patience, because these people were slow and uncoordinated, many had difficulty swallowing and some were regurgitators. The residents in the dining room were expected to feed themselves in any way they could.

Someone approached Rikki and removed her plate, although she had missed some of the food on it. No one had told her what she was eating. Quickly her dinner plate was removed and replaced by a dish of apple sauce. "Excuse me," I said, "but why don't you tell her what she's eating? This resident is blind, and can't see what's on her plate."

The counselor gave me a look of surprise, then disdain. "Gees," she said, "You haven't been here long, have you?"

The food was well-balanced and nutritious, but singularly unappetizing. Sadly, I walked away towards the staff dining room. I stood in the doorway for a few minutes. The odor of food was almost the same, and it was just as noisy, but with the additional strong smell of tobacco smoke. I had completely lost my appetite.

"Anything wrong, Sally?" someone asked. "Come and join us when you've got your tray."

"No, nothing wrong," I said. "Just looking."

* * *

"You can't have food on the wards. It's the rule, Sally," Howard was saying. We were sitting in his office, completing the equipment list. "Food has to be in the dining room. Besides, where would we put dining room furniture?"

"There's plenty of room, Howard," I said. "We can put the beds closer together and have the dining area occupy half the living room. We need the tables for activities anyway. Five square tables and chairs would fit in nicely. We can't teach eating skills in that noisy crowded dining room, and that's an important part of our program."

"And what about the tumbling exercises?" Howard asked. "Where are we going to do that?"

"Our residents have as much right to use the gym as the others, Howard," I responded, "but until we get that arranged we'll just do the mat work in the ward hallway."

"Well, like I said, go ahead and order it," said Howard, "but this has never been done before. All they can do is refuse. I don't think they'll bend the rules that much Sally. You still think you're in a rehab centre. People here don't like that. Take those bars for the toilets now, you won't see any changes made to the washrooms for at least three years. I'll bet my bottom dollar on it. And a bath tub? Forget it! Good grief! Those slabs were put in for safety reasons and efficiency."

"For the staff or for the residents?" I asked. "You know perfectly well they were put there for staff convenience, like everything else here. That's got to change now. That is custodial care thinking. It's out of date. If the staff doesn't want to bend over to wash the tub, then they can teach the residents to do it themselves. It just takes a little more patience, that's all.

"Tell me Howard, how would you like to be hosed down on a slab like an animal? It's undignified. These young blind people don't need that kind of care. We're not dealing with severely retarded people here. Some of these may not even be mentally retarded. They're just blind. Take toilet paper, for instance. I know that some wards don't provide toilet paper because it clogs the toilets. But these residents are capable of learning how to use it, so why not teach them? Just think of the difference in the smell of the ward."

"I know what you're getting at Sally," Howard responded, "but people aren't used to changes here. You can't go too fast. They're used to going by the rules. A place like this has to be run by strict rules, or it gets out of hand. But wait…" Stanley shuffled through the papers on his desk. "…I almost forgot to tell you. There's a memo here. Yes, here it is. The Consultant for the Blind Services from the Government is coming… gee… that's tomorrow. I'll be on leave tomorrow. Do you think you could plan to spend the day with him? Sorry. I guess I should have let you know sooner."

"Of course. I want to meet him anyway. What's his name?"

"Let's see now, oh yes, I've got it here somewhere. Michael something. I don't know if that's his first or his last name. He was here once before, but I was on leave then too. His flight gets in at about eight-thirty. The limo will meet him at the airport. Can you meet him at the front door?"

"Sure Howard, I'll be there."

I sat at my desk in my third floor office, surrounded by books, papers, catalogues, filing folders and memos, trying to decide where to start to prepare for the Consultant tomorrow.

It was just like Howard not to let me know 'til the last minute, and not to be aware that it was important for him to be there too. His priorities were different, he was used to the traditional way of doing things, and he was completely unable to imagine bending the rules or the routine for any reason. There was a singular lack of urgency in his life, established over many years of service in the institution.

Howard had been promoted to his job through seniority. He had grown up through the ranks. Not only did he know everyone, he was related to most of them. He knew the system by heart, and could be relied upon completely to follow it to the letter.

The system was formidable by its inflexible and predictable nature. Everyone was accountable to someone else, so that no one was expected to show any initiative or make original decisions. Even the administrator adhered tenaciously to the system by refusing to speak to anyone who was not immediately next to him in rank, and reporting faithfully to those immediately above him in the government. It was said that he had a great fear of making a mistake or otherwise incurring the displeasure of his superiors. As a result, everything was done by strict rules. Initiative was not rewarded and staff morale was betrayed by an unusually high rate of absenteeism.

In addition to the strict protocol within the custodial system, there was a network of inter-relationship throughout. Entire families were employed here, and anyone concerned about patronage would have a hard time because nearly everyone seemed to be related to everyone else.

I detected a linguistic similarity among the staff, unique to the region, in accent as well as in certain colloquial expressions that made me feel different. When I signed up at Maplegrove I knew that it would mean a long day at a reduced salary, but I wanted the experience. Now I began to wonder if I had done the right thing. Was I really going to be able to work effectively in this environment? Would the Consultant think that I had done enough, or the right things? With no model to follow I would have to use my own judgment all the way, unless the Consultant could help.

I thought again about that motto: "The Impossible Is Only The Untried." Well, here was an opportunity to find out once and for all if that saying was true, because some of the things I wanted to do were already viewed as impossible by most of the staff.

Driving home that night, a CBC host on my car radio was interviewing a well-known Olympic swimmer. When asked the secret of his success he replied, "I never let negative thoughts cloud my thinking."

I decided to try to adopt that motto too.

Chapter 11

POWER AND PURPOSE

"Men are wise in proportion, not to their experience, but to their capacity for experience."
George Bernard Shaw

My spirit of optimism for the new ward was contagious to a certain degree, but every step closer to the goal of opening the ward had been challenged by administrative hurdles and a certain amount of skepticism from the staff, particularly from those who were only indirectly involved. I made every effort to disguise any misgivings I had and depended on the Government's support for my actions, in spite of the fact that "the Government", up to this time had been a phantom, with all the power and no face.

While I feared that I had not accomplished anything really tangible during the past few weeks, because everything was still only on paper, I welcomed the visit of the Consultant to support our program to give me advice on how to proceed. I wondered if he would be pleased with our progress, or if he would be unduly critical and hard to work with.

I arrived at Maplegrove the next morning with feelings of both apprehension and excitement. The large entrance hall looked like any hospital lobby except that it was deserted. I was the only one there. The marble floor glistened where the morning sun shone through the heavy double glass doors, and reflected the colours from large urns of flowers that decorated the lobby. There were no chairs or benches, so I paced back and forth across the area, aware that my footsteps sounded unnaturally loud in the silence, and thinking what a contrast this attractive lobby was to the bleakness of the wards.

When a black limousine drew up to the door I watched the uniformed driver get out and walk around to assist the passenger. My first surprise was that this was a woman, not a man as I had expected. Then I noticed that the woman was carrying a white cane that she had just unfolded from her purse.

Dr. Mikaela Piercey was a smartly dressed, attractive woman in her mid-thirties. Long blond hair was neatly drawn back into a chignon, enhancing regular features, fair complexion, and not much make-up. She wore dark glasses.

"Please call me Mikaela," Dr. Piercey was saying as she took my arm and we began the long walk down the main corridor. "How long have you been here? How many staff do you have now? I would like to meet all the prospective residents individually while I'm here."

I felt at ease with Mikaela immediately, and also stimulated. Her questions were direct and penetrating. Her professional manner gave the impression of strength, assurance, and scrutiny.

"I'll be here for two days," Mikaela was saying. "Reservations were made for me at a local motel. Can you make yourself available during this time? I'd like you to accompany me to assess all the visually impaired who have any potential for this ward, and to meet all the staff and review the programming. I would like to see the ward open next week."

"Next week? I was alarmed. "But we're not nearly ready! We haven't got the furniture yet, except for the beds."

"Never mind," Mikaela said quietly. "This is the way to get it."

The staff had been alerted to be ready for a meeting shortly after nine o'clock. The meeting went well. Initial reserve gave way to heated discussion, everything from short biographies of prospective clients to attitudes, training methods, blindisms, and normalization.

"You must all be very verbal," Mikaela was saying. "Use all your skills to put across an idea, and then provide feed-back so that the resident learns by immediate reinforcement, not the "Behavior Modification" type of reward, like Smarties, that won't work with this type of resident, but with the knowledge that he has done the required thing correctly because it has achieved the desired result. The activity must have meaning to him. Putting a peg into a board has no meaning, but pressing a lever to turn on a tape recorder does have meaning and gives the immediate desired result. Do you understand what I mean?"

"But... what if he doesn't understand language and doesn't talk?" asked one of the counselors.

"It doesn't matter. A baby learns this way, doesn't he? You don't wait 'til he understands language before you talk to him. He learns by listening, and then, by trial and error, developing his own code of language, not copying yours. But it's very important for him to get an immediate consistent response, and you may find that repetition is necessary to a certain extent. Remember that blind people can't see your facial expression, so you must let him know your reaction in another way." The staff listened intently as Mikaela continued. This was not theorizing, it was meaningful down-to-earth information about how to proceed, and as we sat in the little office I felt the excitement in the air.

Mikaela continued. "Go slowly, but consistently. Look first at the skills they already have. Can they walk, sit, vocalize? These are the basic skills we have to build on. Introduce new ideas gradually, and take the time to let the residents do certain things for themselves. Don't do it for them. Start with daily living skills and work from there. For example, finding their way around, decide where the furniture is to go, then don't move it without showing the residents the changes. If you move a chair out from the table, put it back the way it was, and teach them to do the same. You're not just counselors now, you are also teachers."

"Sally has asked for dining room furniture on the ward," said Howard. "Do you think the Ministry will approve that? It's never...."

"Of course, Howard," replied Mikaela. "This would be an important part of the training program. You know the procedure. Send the requisition in to my department, not by the regular channels, but justify your reasons for needing it and it will be dealt with immediately. We don't want undue delay with this project. If you have an order ready before I leave I'll take it."

"Does that mean things like Braille watches?" asked Darlene.

"There are better ways to teach concept of time Darlene, at this stage," said Mikaela, "but eventually, yes, anything you need for your program. Braille is premature for your residents, except for one or possibly two. What you need initially are remedial adult-type learning materials and equipment. Sally will know the sort of things. They are designed to teach concepts of spatial awareness, distance judgment, body image. Your people will be lacking all those skills. Sighted people take them for granted, but blind people have to be taught. Remember, they only know what they can feel, taste, hear and smell, unless you teach them."

"What about white canes?" asked Darlene. "When should we introduce them?"

"You'll have to try to get an Orientation and Mobility instructor from the Agency for the Blind to help you with that," replied Mikaela. "The two go hand in hand. Just for now, try to teach them to orient themselves by sound and touch cues, like learning to trail the back of their hand along the wall, or feeling the change in floor texture with their feet. If you reduce noise in the ward to meaningful sound cues, like a radio or television or a clock, they'll learn where it is. Teach them to find their way to the bathroom, the cloakroom and their beds. They'll soon learn, if there are no unexpected obstacles in the way."

I could not remember ever spending a more exciting or satisfying day. I dropped Mikaela off at her motel on her way home and arranged to pick her up at eight-thirty the next morning. She appeared to be indefatigable. Her mind seemed to work like the proverbial steel trap. She gave the impression that she remembered every word that was said. She seemed more astute than anyone I had ever met, and now we had someone to help us.

I was tired, but elated. Mikaela had given me the confidence and support that I needed. I marveled at how much we had accomplished in one day. Now I could hardly wait for tomorrow.

Chapter 12

MAYBE THERE WILL BE COFFEE

"What can be immediately accomplished is always questionable, and what can be finally accomplished, inconceivable."
John Ruskin

Mikaela was ready and waiting at the motel door when I drew up. On the way to Maplegrove, she outlined the plan for the day, and I wondered how we would ever accomplish it all. While Mikaela had a word with the Administrator, Mr. Charles Nash, I informed Claire, in my own department, of my plans for the day. First on the agenda was a meeting with Dr. Peter Ambrose, Chief of Medical Services. I had met Dr. Ambrose on several occasions, but never for any lengthy discussion. He always seemed to be too busy, so I welcomed this opportunity.

The secretary ushered us into a comfortable office. It had thick pale green carpet, shelves of medical books on the walls, brown leather furniture, contemporary painting reproductions, homespun curtains, and a picture window looked out over spacious, well-kept lawns. Dr. Ambrose rose from behind his desk and held out his hand.

"Dr. Ambrose," Mikaela began, after the usual preliminaries, "I'm impressed with the organization of this new ward as far as it goes, but I'd like to see the first residents phasing in by Monday. Do you see that as a possibility?"

His smile altered to one of uncertainty. "Well... yes... indeed, we would like to see it go ahead, of course..."

"We will need your complete cooperation," continued Mikaela. "The Government will supply the equipment and furniture on a high priority basis. What are your feelings about the program so far?"

I began to feel uncomfortable. Dr. Ambrose had not attended any of the ward meetings, and I was uncertain how much he actually knew because all reports went through department heads and unit directors to the Administrator.

"I saw the list of proposed residents, Dr. Piercey. "It appears that the higher functioning and younger residents are to be moved first. I assume that they're the best candidates for training. You obviously feel that more can be done for them on a special ward."

Dr. Ambrose altered his position, looked out the window for a moment, and then continued, "You may not be aware, however, that one or two of our doctors, and some of the parents too, are not at all in favour of this segregation of the blind. In fact they are against it, particularly the proposed co-ed arrangement. Tell me, what do you expect to ultimately achieve by this special program? We have lots of special programs, you know, such as the summer volunteers, and the Chaplain's music program..."

"Dr. Piercey can reply to that with regard to the government proposals, Dr. Ambrose," I replied, "but essentially we're trying to provide a more normal environment to make it easier for them to learn."

Dr. Piercey added, "The ministry plan is based on the advice of experts in the field, Dr. Ambrose. We know that all people learn by sensory stimulation; vision, hearing, taste, smell, touch, balance - and if any of these receptors is missing the others have to compensate. In the case of blindness, the person is dependent mainly on hearing, touch, balance and position sense, and to a lesser degree on the other senses.

"A high noise level on the ward, continual pushing, punching, walking into furniture and other forms of "punishment", result in a hostile environment, causing a blind person to retreat into himself for protection. If the messages he gets are contradictory, he may actually appear to be retarded when he may not be, or develop deviant behavior patterns, like abusing himself or striking out at others. The government is concerned about the large number of sensory impaired individuals residing in our institutions, who have had no training programs directed towards alleviating the problems of hearing or vision loss. I understand that most of the counselors assigned to this special ward volunteered to come, but they were also chosen for their ability and enthusiasm and are probably the best we could have found for this program."

"Are you saying that some of these people may not actually be retarded, Dr Piercey?"

"That's a possibility. But years of living in an institutional environment will take some time to reverse, because the blind residents in particular, have been deprived of programs to meet their special needs, and that's one of the ministry's main concerns. We wish to introduce appropriate programs for these specific needs."

"I see." Dr. Ambrose leaned back in his chair and thought for a minute. "You will, of course, have met with Mr. Nash, the Administrator?" Dr. Piercey nodded. "Yes, well... I appreciate your keeping me informed. I'll be happy to help all I can."

The interview was over. Mikaela took my arm as we walked down the corridor towards the new ward.

"I'd like to speak to the ward supervisor to arrange the interviews for this afternoon," she said. "Let's see if he's in his office." I explained that Howard was away on leave.

"Well then, we'll just go to the wards. I want to see Chrissie, Rory and Harry first, and Peer too, and I'd like to meet your protégé, Rikki Chase. A pity she's in a wheelchair and can't be part of the new ward, but I agree with the decision about that. Perhaps I can help you create something else for Rikki."

While most of the candidates for the new ward were scattered throughout the institution, Chrissie, Rory and Harry had been together on ward A for many years. All the wards were laid out in the same way. The door from the Unit corridor led into a windowless hallway, with three or four rooms on either side and the open ward ahead. On the right, were the doctors' examining office, the ward supervisor's office, the washing room, with its metal slab and shower hose, large basins and laundry containers, and then the ward office, with a large picture window looking into the ward. On the left of the corridor were the clothing rooms and the residents' toilets; five cubicles without doors and five wash basins.

On entering from the corridor the senses of hearing and smell were immediately assailed. The sound could only be properly described as noise. The smell was like a stable smell, only human, with a strong odor of urine near the toilets.

The ward supervisor told us that Chrissie and Harry were sitting in their usual place on the couch. Rory was wandering around at the back of the ward, and Peer was out for a haircut and would be back soon. Mikaela asked if there were any other blind residents on this ward. The supervisor replied that he did not know. He had only been assigned here a few months ago. He described Chrissie and Harry as "easy-care" residents, because they were content to sit and rock back and forth on the couch most of the day. Rory was always complaining about something. Peer was a different matter, but we would see that for ourselves.

Chrissie's most distinguishing feature was his thick dark curly hair. He was a slender boy of fifteen, whose limbs seemed to have grown too fast for his body. Early records about Chrissie were incomplete. He had been admitted to Maplegrove at the age of five from an orphanage in Middleton that had been closed. Efforts to trace his parents had been unsuccessful.

I was intrigued by Mikaela's approach to Chrissie. Taking the boy firmly by both hands, she raised him to his feet, tucked one arm through her own, and proceeded to walk with him about the ward, talking as they went. I wondered how Mikaela knew where she was going, but assumed that she had enough vision to see the essentials. Mikaela established a relationship with Chrissie immediately, and he was responding. Back again at the couch, Mikaela turned to Harry.

I thought that Harry was too handsome to be retarded. He was obviously of European, possibly Slavic descent. Dark eyebrows and eyelashes matched the straight black hair, cut in a classic fashion. As a young child it was thought that Harry showed some autistic characteristics, but as he grew older he became more sociable and obedient. Harry was admitted to Maplegrove at the age of seven, following the death of his father in an industrial accident. At that time Harry spoke no English, was totally blind, and had never been toilet trained. He did not do well on the admission tests and was assumed to be severely retarded. He was now seventeen years old. Harry was big for his age, but he lacked the muscular control and coordination of a normal seventeen year old. There was a softness about him that indicated lack of muscle tone.

"Tell me something about yourself, Harry," said Mikaela, holding him by the hand. "How old are you?

"Don't know. Quite old, I think. Are you going to work here?"

"No. I'm just visiting, Harry. My name is Mikaela."

"That's nice. I'm Harry. I'm going to a new ward."

"Do you want to go to the new ward?"

"Yes, I do."

"Why?"

"Because Sally said I should go. Sally is very smart. She said I should go."

"What do you think it will be like there?"

"Oh, it will be nice. Maybe there will be coffee."

"Don't you have coffee here?"

"On Sundays we have coffee."

"Show me what you can do, Harry." Mikaela helped him to his feet, but instead of walking around the ward, as she had done with Chrissie, Mikaela asked him to get up and down from the floor, identify objects, stand on one foot, and clap his hands in rhythm.

While Mikaela was working with Harry, Chrissie had returned to his favourite pastime of rocking back and forth, paying no attention to what was going on.

"This rocking is a "blindism", explained Mikaela. "It should be discouraged, but it can't be done in a hurry. A long-established habit like this can't be altered overnight without undesirable side-effects, so don't let the staff push it. Diversion is the best tactic."

While we were talking, one of the counselors brought Rory to meet us. He was a gaunt, unhappy looking young man in his late twenties, with poor rather stooped posture. He kept wringing his hands together accentuating his nervousness. Mikaela stepped forward and took Rory's right hand in both of hers, introducing herself at the same time.

"I hope we can become friends, Rory. I hear that you're coming on the new ward."

"Oh, I don't know M'am," said Rory, pronouncing his words slowly, "I don't know if I can. My stomach hurts something awful today, and I had a pain in my leg last night."

"Rory always has lots of aches and pains, Dr Piercey," said the counselor. "We've had him checked over, but he seems OK. The pains just come and go, don't they, Rory?"

We returned to the staff room where we discussed programming for Chrissie, Harry and Rory with several counselors over a cup of coffee and waited for Peer to return to the ward. The name Peer was derived from Pierre, invented by the staff with no knowledge of French. Peer quickly lost any French he might have known and learned English, and his family gradually lost contact.

Peer was admitted at age six. His family was working class, without much education. They felt embarrassed about having a disabled child. At first his father tried to convince him that he could see if he tried hard enough. He had no patience with what he called Peer's ineptitude, and Peer became an abused child. He was removed from the home for his own protection. Test scores at Maplegrove, as with all the blind residents, indicated below normal intelligence, although Peer possessed, even at that time, two qualities that set him apart from the other boys. He was aggressive, with a quick temper, and he had good verbal skills.

As Peer entered the ward and cautiously felt his way along, feeling the wall with the back of his hand, Mikaela remarked that he already had the basis of good mobility skills. Peer was now eighteen and big for his age, with a shock of brick-red hair and a mass of freckles. I thought he had a very Irish face.

"Get out of my way!" Peer shouted to a resident who crossed his path.

"Peer! You cut that out!" one of the staff barked back. Peer continued to make his way through the ward towards his bed in one of the two sunrooms at the far end of the ward. Mikaela and I followed and waited until he was seated on the side of his bed.

"Hello Peer", I said. "May we come in? I want you to meet Mikaela, our consultant from the government who has come to see us."

"Hello Mikaela…" asked Peer in a belligerent tone of voice.

"I don't see very well either, Peer. Did you get a nice haircut?"

"Can you get me out of here?" asked Peer, ignoring her question.

"Maybe, Peer. The first step is to get you over to the new ward."

"O.K. I'm going. I already know all that junk. These people don't know anything. They're all stupid. I want out of here."

"Where would you go, Peer?"

"To the city. There's lots of work there. I want to do some work. They won't let you do anything here. All you do is sit around."

"What kind of work could you do Peer?" asked Mikaela. "Tell me about it."

"All kinds. I'm a good worker. Just let me try."

"That's a good attitude, but you have to develop skills first. What sort of skills do you have?"

"I just want to be able to do some work so that I can be tired when I go to sleep at night. And I want to learn how to read. One of the volunteers showed me some of that stuff called Braille. I could learn that."

"Perhaps you could," said Mikaela. "Do you think we could have Peer tested by the Agency for the Blind, Sally? Why not invite them to come out when the new ward is opened?"

The interviews became more difficult as the day progressed. Ginny, the only blind resident on a ward for disturbed residents, had just had a temper tantrum and was "on punishment", having ripped her clothing and thrown a drinking glass across the room. Ginny was described as "self abusive". Her blindness had been self-inflicted in a fit of temper. Residents who were "on punishment" were confined in a room by themselves for a certain period of time.

Charlie was a tall, dark haired young man who looked under-nourished. He was described as being "echolalic", meaning that he never initiated any language himself; his speech was only a parrot-like repetition of what someone else had just said. Looking at the many scratches and bruises on his thin body, I suspected that he too was self-abusive, but the ward supervisor assured us that he was not.

"The problem is with the other guys," the supervisor explained. "Charlie can't see where he's going, and when he walks into someone he gets beaten up. They're all aggressive on this ward. They don't understand that he can't see. We can't do anything about it. The sooner he's moved the better for him, that's what I say."

Donny was fourteen but he looked like a seven year old. He was obviously the favourite on his ward, and I suspected that the staff was reluctant to let him go. Donny had his own method of communication that sounded like a chipmunk. He could get an idea across without using any conventional language. The staff would pick him up and rock him like a baby and tickle him to make him laugh. Donny was well proportioned except for a rather large head, the result of hydrocephalus that was controlled with a shunt.

It was hard to find time for Mikaela to meet Rikki, but I felt that I could not let Mikaela go without some advice about Rikki's program, partly for my own information and partly to impress the staff with its importance for her.

"She's very alert," said Mikaela after meeting Rikki. "You're right that she needs to get off the ward every day somehow. It's a pity she can't go to the schoolroom any more. Keep trying to get "Talking Books" and a cassette player for her. It's too much for you to be making all those tapes.

It had been a long day. I felt saturated with information, but I was reluctant to let Mikaela go before asking every possible question.

"You have a good start now," Mikaela was saying. "Phone me at my office any time you like. I could come again in about a month if you want me. Now, I want you to think about something else. I would like you to prepare a seminar for three months from now, to be held here, for all the other provincial institutions, so that they can see what you're doing."

I was speechless. Then, "A seminar? Us? You've got to be kidding! We're nowhere near ready....."

"You will be. Don't worry about it. I'll help you. But tell the staff now. I'll make the arrangements with Mr. Nash. I feel that it's very important for the staff from all the institutions to share their ideas and to learn from each other, and not to be pioneers all working in isolation."

At four o'clock I walked with Mikaela to the front entrance where the driver was waiting to take her to the airport.

"Any problems, Sally, just give me a call. Don't allow yourself to be pushed, though. Move those first three boys in on Monday. Keep them together, then phase in the others, two by two, as you're ready. It won't hurt to have only three the first week. Then it will start getting easier. And start right in with rehab. methods. You're going to have to train the staff as much as the residents at first, and the results will act as reinforcers."

"I wish I had your confidence, Mikaela. It's been a great experience having you here. You've been a great help."

I suddenly felt overwhelmed with exhaustion, yet Mikaela appeared as fresh as when she arrived.

I think I'm going to learn just as much as the residents, I thought, as I turned towards my department to write my reports and make preparations for the weekend. I was right.

Chapter 13

WE CAN DO ANYTHING

"What we anticipate seldom occurs; what we least expect generally happens."
Benjamin Disraeli

One thing that I learned in my first month at Maplegrove was not to expect anything to go exactly as planned. On the other hand, I also learned that the word of the Government was law, and must be carried out to the letter. The efforts of the staff to make a good impression on Mikaela did not go unnoticed by me. Yet, in fairness to the staff, their energy and enthusiasm had obviously made a good impression.

Upon my arrival that Monday morning, I was greeted on Ward B with a hum of activity preparing to welcome the first three residents, in spite of a delay in finishing the bathroom for the girls. The beds had arrived and were being arranged with suitable spacing between each. Two firm leather chesterfields and several easy chairs were being carried in and put in place.

Howard Sylvester, being the most senior person on the ward, was busy arranging papers on his desk, calling out instructions, answering the telephone and generally trying to do many things at once. He was a kind, friendly man in his mid-thirties, tall, easy-going, with a soft voice, liked and respected by the staff. Darlene began making up the beds with clean sheets and brightly coloured bedspreads. She had even located bolts of bright woven material from the handicraft shop for curtains for the windows. There had never been curtains on wards but Mikaela had stressed the importance of bright colours for the low-vision residents. All were legally blind but not all of them were totally blind. It was important for those with low vision to use what they had as much as possible.

Darlene was the youngest staff member, not very experienced, cautious, yet willing to learn. She was a pretty girl, with short bobbed fair hair, fair complexion and dark eyes.

"Oh, so you're here Sally." said Howard, as I entered the office. "There's a call for you on line two. You can take it in here."

The call was from Rikki's ward. The supervisor wanted to see me immediately about a problem with Rikki. "I'm going down to ward C, Howard," I said. "I'll be back shortly."

Three of the ward C staff were waiting for me in the office.

"We thought we'd better have a word with you, Sally," said Yvonne, the supervisor. "Rikki has thrown another of her tantrums this morning. She won't do anything she's told, and keeps saying that you said she doesn't have to. Maybe we should have a case conference and get our goals straightened out."

"That's a good idea, Yvonne. As you know, I've been busy on the other ward, and haven't had time for Rikki the last few days. What's the problem today?"

"It's mostly her attitude. She thinks she's better than the others, and today she bit Carmel on the arm. Rikki and

Carmel are always fighting, and Rikki won't cooperate with the staff. Mabel, here, is trying to teach her colours and how to tie her shoe laces, and Rikki won't even try. If she's so damn smart she ought to be able to learn those things."

"I see the problem, Yvonne," I said. "You see, Rikki *is* smarter than the others on this ward, but she has cerebral palsy. This affects her motor ability and her sense of touch, but not her intelligence. She should not be telling you that I said she doesn't have to do it, but she knows that *I* know she can't. She has no position sense or normal feeling in her left hand, and she can't use her right hand at all. It's like asking you to tie shoe laces with only one hand, with a glove on it so you can't feel the laces, and your eyes shut. It can't be done. Just try it. And you can't teach colours with plastic shapes, Yvonne. Why don't you read to her instead?"

"We haven't time for that," said Mabel. "Have you any idea of the work that has to be done on this ward? Only four staff and..."

"Yes, I know, Mabel. I'm going to try to get Rikki off the ward every day for awhile. That will relieve you quite a bit and will give Rikki an outlet."

"Gee, I don't know about that," said Yvonne. "That's not really fair to the other residents, you know. It looks like Rikki's getting preferential treatment. We try to treat them all alike. Besides, I don't know where you can take her. Every available space is occupied."

"I understand what you're saying, Yvonne, and I'm sorry if it causes problems. But Rikki is the only blind resident on this ward, and I've been hired specially to work with the blind. That includes Rikki, and she needs a special program. Then she'll be easier on the ward."

"Are you saying there's something wrong with our program?" asked Bernice, angrily. "We've already set the goals for Rikki for the next six months. What are *you* going to do with her? That's the trouble with all you people coming in from outside and starting special programs. It just causes a lot of trouble."

"This is different, Bernice. It's under the direction of the Government. And Rikki needs a program that can't be offered on the ward. Because of her blindness, she must be in a quiet place so that she can use her hearing better. Then she needs to be taught many of the things sighted people take for granted. As I said earlier, she needs to be read to. She needs cognitive training, not motor training. We do need a conference, because it's important that we work together with Rikki, and that you understand what I'm doing with her. Just for now, though, forget the shoe laces. I'll help you work out some goals that she can do within the limits of her motor ability."

Rikki was sobbing in the corner of the sunroom. "Oh Sally," she cried, "they're all crackers in here except me, including the staff. They're mean too. And I hate that Carmel. She comes and pushes my chair and I tell her to stop, and she won't, and she calls me names and won't go away."

"All right Rikki, I've heard all about it. Now I want you to turn off the water-works and listen to me closely. Right now! You and I know something no one else knows on this ward, right?"

"What?" asked Rikki through her tears.

"You know that you're smart enough to go out to a group home. You know you have normal intelligence. Right? O.K., I want you to use it. Stop letting Carmel tease you. She only does it because it gets a rise out of you. Stop reacting so much. Flatter her a bit. It only makes Carmel worse by reacting the way you do. And you must not tell the staff that I said you don't need to do things. You did that at rehab too, and it only makes trouble for me, and that's not fair. That puts me in a bad position with the staff."

"But they want..."

"Yes, I know. They don't understand C.P. Well, we'll deal with that. In the meantime, you try to do what they ask as well as you can, until I can get a program going for you."

"Sally, may I ask you a question?"

"Of course Rikki."

There was silence for a moment. Rikki took a deep breath. "Why did they turn me down for the group home?"

I thought for a moment. "I know why they *said* they turned you down, but I don't think that was the real reason. I was not on the selection committee. I only know that they had a lot of applications, so they had to take what they thought were the best or most deserving candidates. One reason may have been that Owen House was planned as a group home for physically disabled adults from Rehab. who had no place to go. It was not intended as a home for blind people. It's the same old problem, Rikki. The Agency for the Blind won't take you because you have cerebral palsy. That's why you're here, and this isn't right for you either."

"But I was promised. They said that the house was started for me, and my parents even went to the meeting."

"Yes, I know." I thought for a moment. "I can think of many reasons, Rikki. They said that you were not independent enough. Do you think that was the reason?"

"No. They already knew what I could do when they started planning the house."

"Yes. So that was not the real reason. I think it was something else. But never mind. We've had a few set-backs before, and what did I tell you? I said we weren't giving up, didn't I? We're not quitters. So they refused you. Well, we've just got to work harder, that's all."

"Sally, You're my very best friend in the whole world. Together I guess we can do anything."

"Hey, that's the spirit I like to see."

During the next few days Chrissie, Peer, Rory and Harry began adjusting to the new ward, and the staff enjoyed having plenty of time to spend with them.

"I like listening to the silence," said Harry one day. I noticed that Chrissie was not spending as much time rocking. Peer was delighted with his new bed and he had been promised a big box with a lock on it that he could keep under his bed to hold his own possessions.

The staff worked out methods to teach dressing, teeth brushing and feeding techniques. They played games with the residents, like passing bean bags from one to another, leading to teaching the boys to pass plates at the table. These activities were also teaching concepts of sharing, awareness of each other and assuming some responsibility for themselves and others.

Charlie and Donny were introduced to the ward the next day.

"You won't believe how easily they've fitted in, Sally," Darlene was saying. "Donny is such a cutie. It's a wonder F ward parted with him. He looks so much younger than he is. I can see why they tended to spoil him. He can't say anything you can understand, but he gets the idea across."

"What about Charlie?" I asked. "He had some behavior problems I believe?"

"Good as gold, and quite intelligent, I think. Rory's not very happy yet, though. He always has an ache or pain somewhere, it may take awhile to change that."

The dining room furniture arrived that afternoon, much to everyone's surprise. It was almost unheard of to receive an order so quickly. There were five square tables with matching captain's chairs, in red maple. We had particularly wanted square tables so that the blind residents could locate themselves by the corners. Chrissie went from one table to another, feeling the smooth satin finish. Darlene was helping him, teaching him to count them as he moved along. Each person was given his own special place at the tables and meal time became an enjoyable experience. The boys soon learned that no one was going to steal their food. Forks were introduced along with spoons and plate guards were produced where necessary. The staff devised tricks with the food, like gluing peas together with mashed potatoes.

"How is the exercise program progressing," I asked one morning.

"It was really funny today," said Darlene. "Chrissie found out where his head was, and none of them knew how to reach out to the side. They really enjoy it. We're keeping track of all the skills on a big chart. Want to see it?"

"Why that's marvelous, Darlene," I said. "Did you make that? Just look at the progress they've made already."

I was impressed with the ideas and motivation of the staff and I enjoyed seeing how they responded to the results they were getting. Staff morale had never been so high. It was high among the residents too. They were becoming like a family, and everyone was impressed with how they were beginning to talk among themselves, something that was never expected on the other wards.

But there was no time to become complacent, because changes occurred every day and the following week something happened to suggest another change needed for the new ward.

It was about three-fifteen in the afternoon. I had finished my reports and had decided to drop in to see Rikki for awhile before going home. On entering the ward I could hardly believe my eyes. I was astounded to see that all the residents on the ward were stark naked. All the beds had been stripped too, and not a piece of clothing was to be seen anywhere.

"What is going on?" I asked. Two counselors were writing at the desk while a third was apportioning out medication into little paper cups on a tray. No one looked up.

"There's nothing the matter," one replied, in a bored tone. "It's *strip day*, that's all. Kelly has the key to the cupboards and she hasn't come in yet. She'll be in soon. The laundry has to go in by three o'clock."

I was angry. "But this is an indignity to the residents," I said. "It's not decent. How would *you* like to be treated like that?"

"Oh come on, Sally," said Mabel. "They're used to it. We've got our job to do. If you worked on this ward you'd soon see what it's like. We haven't time to think about modesty in an institution like this, and they don't know the difference anyway."

Rikki was sitting in her wheelchair at the back of the ward. I looked around. What a variety of shapes the human body could assume, and what cruelty and injustice to the human form. There were pretty faces with misshapen bodies, and beautiful bodies with ugly faces. Small women weighed down by huge breasts, short women with huge abdomens, frail skeleton-like figures with pinched faces - all helpless, trusting, existing, with no cure, no hope - pathetic human sheep. I felt both sad and angry as I walked back to my ward. Darlene was still on duty.

"How do you keep track of the clothing, Darlene?" I asked.

"What do you mean, Sally? It's all labeled. It's kept in the cupboard."

"Do you have "strip day" on this ward?"

"Well, we do have laundry day. It's not quite like the other wards. We put clean linen on the beds once a week."

"Can the residents select their clothing themselves?"

"No. How would they do that?"

"Suppose they all had their own dressers? They could learn to look after their own clothing."

"Oh, we'd never be allowed to do that."

"Why not?"

"My Gosh, Sally, you're the limit! Why not, eh? Well, I don't know. Are you going to ask?"

"If you think it's a good idea," I said.

The following week three young women, all in their early twenties, joined the ranks of the blind boys on ward B. Ginny Craig settled in quite well, considering her previous behavior record. It was decided to give her a chance, to see if the acting-out behavior would be reduced in the new environment.

Molly Allen's voice could be heard all over the ward, and staff and residents alike had to keep reminding her that she no longer had to shout to be heard. Vivianne Dean had been selected with some misgivings because of her bouts of depression, but she seemed to have intelligence underneath the mood swings and it seemed appropriate to give her a chance too. More staff were introduced as the number of residents increased. The original counselors were given the more senior positions, and they were able to arrange to be on permanent day shift, with part-time staff taking over evening duty. Fewer staff were required for night duty because our residents were sleeping well and there were few behavior problems.

One day I dropped into the cafeteria for a short break and found Philip Martin there. "I hear great reports about the progress of your new ward Sally," said Philip. "Are you happy with the results so far?"

"Oh yes, Philip," I replied. "The Government has been great, and staff morale couldn't be better."

"Has Mr. Nash been down to see the program on the ward?"

"Not while I've been there, Philip. Isn't that strange? I thought he'd be more interested."

"Well, he's an odd one. Doesn't really like the project, you know. He doesn't like change at all. But he's afraid to go against the Government."

"You'd think he would want to encourage a thing like this. What's he so afraid of? Why doesn't he like it?" I asked.

"Several reasons, I think," replied Philip. "He hasn't been getting any favourable feed-back from some of the senior staff, particularly the psychologists, and he gets most of his information from the heads of departments. That's why he doesn't talk to you. It doesn't necessarily mean that he doesn't like the program, but you'd be surprised to know how many people come here with innovative ideas, and they just get started and then the key people leave and everything reverts back to where it was. It's a common problem with big institutions. That's probably the main reason why he's suspicious of change."

"One thing I can't understand, Philip," I said. "is why we haven't had any psychologists assigned to our ward. I thought they, especially, would be interested in this program, but one actually sent me a note saying that he disagreed too much with what we were doing to have any part in it. We had invited him to a ward meeting.

"You know why that happened, Sally? They don't want to be part of it unless they're running it, and they don't know anything about working with blind residents. Look at how they've been testing them!"

"I guess you're right." I said. "Too bad. But I still think it's strange that Mr. Nash wouldn't have wanted to see what we're doing. You'd think he'd try to encourage something that seems to be working and is requested by the Government."

"Yes, I agree Sally, but you're not hired through the usual channels, you see, so he doesn't really trust you. People like you never stay. It's because you don't really come under the authority of anyone except the Government, and your department. You admit yourself that your department head doesn't know what you're doing either."

"She knows, but she doesn't really understand. She's very busy with the other areas, and doesn't have much interest in the blind. Her background is all in psychiatry and mental retardation."

"So your independence is either an asset or a hindrance, depending on how you look at it. Come to my office tomorrow and we'll go over the list and see who should be phased in next."

I sensed a certain reserve on the part of the professional staff in other departments, and decided that perhaps I should make an effort to meet them and not wait for them to come to see me. Apart from Philip, no one had made any particular effort to talk to me, so I decided that they were waiting for me to make the first move. I knew that there was only one physiotherapist on staff and one speech pathologist. I wondered how they would ever decide who to treat among sixteen hundred residents.

I had always worked closely with the physiotherapists at Rehab. I decided to pay a visit to the physiotherapy department tomorrow.

Chapter 14

HITTING THE WALL

"The prevailing wind shapes the pine."
Birnie Hodgetts

The first day of November was dark, wet, and gloomy as I arrived at the institution. There were now fifteen residents on the new ward, now called Special B with ten men and five women, an average age of twenty-one. Many were congenitally blind, caused by a condition called retrolental fibroplasia, the result of premature birth and high concentrations of oxygen. Some had been rubella babies, and one boy had self-inflicted blindness and schizophrenia. Some had very low vision. All had an additional disability, physical or behavioral, that limited their ability to learn and develop in a normal way.

There were now eight counselors on Special B, in addition to the team, including Dr. Ambrose and Philip Martin. After Dr Piercey's visit, Dr. Ambrose began to show a real interest in the project, dropping in almost every day. He was there this day when I arrived, and held the door for me.

"I thought I would just pop in again Sally, he asked. How is everything progressing?"

"Quite well Doctor. Something new happens every day. The electric razors arrived yesterday and we're teaching the boys to use them. All the tooth brushes are marked in some way now, and the towel racks, and they're each getting to know their own mark. We haven't had any behavior problems, except for Ginny. She has periods of being good, and then she suddenly throws her dinner plate across the room. This morning she didn't want to get out of bed."

"But you're going to keep trying with her, are you? Yes, well that's good. I wanted to ask you about something else. Have you ever had any experience with horseback riding for disabled people? Such programs have been very successful in England and Europe, and I just thought it might be possible. There's a small stable with an arena only about five miles from here."

"What a tremendous idea," I said. Because I had been a rider and horse owner for many years, I knew about such programs for handicapped people. "Would there be funding for such a program for our residents?"

"I should imagine it would come out of the Program budget," replied Dr. Ambrose. "The Ministry is quite receptive to innovative programs for this ward... if you think it would be beneficial, of course."

"It's a great idea, Dr. Ambrose," I responded. I immediately thought of all the fringe benefits, like getting the residents outdoors, teaching them about animals, and providing the necessary exercise and stimulation. "I'll call the stable today."

Later that morning I went up to ward F to see two other candidates for Special B, Tony and Colin, who had not been moved yet. Like many of the blind residents, they both looked younger than they were. They were in their early twenties, but looked more like sixteen-year-olds. I found them in the sunroom at the back of the ward, sitting on a piano bench at an old Heinzman piano. Tony was running his fingers over the keys, but there was no sound.

"Play something for me, Tony," I asked.

"Can't," replied Tony.

"Oh, come on. Don't be shy. Just play anything."

"Can't," replied Tony again.

"Can you play something, Colin?"

"Nope."

"Well then, move over and let me try," I said, taking Tony's place. To my surprise, the piano was completely mute. Not a sound came forth.

I entered the ward office. Two counselors were busy writing at the desk. "About that piano..." I said. No one looked up. "Who's in charge here?"

"Carla," said one of the staff. "She's off on break."

"Well, who can I talk to about the piano?"

"What about it?"

"It doesn't work."

"So what else is new? Nothing works here except us."

"Well, what good is it?" I persisted. "Why don't you get it fixed ?"

"Because it would just get broken again. What's the point? And there's enough noise on this ward anyway."

I wandered about the ward, waiting for Carla to return. This ward was no different from all the others. It might have been a kind of zoo, except that the inmates were people, people with nothing to do, so that what they did instead was a form of escape, mostly meaningless, some of it self-stimulating or even injurious. One boy kept slapping his own face over and over, his cheek becoming redder with each slap. Eventually he smiled. Another held a piece of glitter above his head and peered at it intently as he moved it with his hand to make it shine. Another was curled up on the floor in the corner of the room in a fetal position, arms and legs interwoven, head down. Many were shouting, screaming or singing.

Carla agreed to part with the piano when I said that I would like to have it for Special B. It was an easy matter to have it picked up and repaired by Maintenance, and then moved into the new ward.

I was in daily contact with Claire, and tried to keep her informed about my work, but Claire was too busy to talk for long at a time. She was chief of a department of twenty, mostly occupational therapy aids. The three occupational therapists worked in different areas of the institution and I seldom saw them. Many of the aids worked in handicraft departments such as weaving, art, pottery and woodworking. There were actually several members of my department that I had never met.

As time went by, I gradually met other professionals, but the building was so huge, with such a large population, that it was like a city in itself. While there were sixteen hundred residents at this time, as well as about the same number of staff, there was nothing like a one-to-one ratio of staff to resident. This was because large segments of staff administered only to staff, some worked in maintenance, some in engineering and grounds, some in the food and kitchen department, laundry and cleaning, and there was a large secretarial and business administration staff.

There were many unit staff in the institution who never saw the residents. As they became supervisors and rose within the hierarchy they gradually lost direct care responsibilities. While I saw no evidence of active physiotherapy as I had known it in hospitals or rehabilitation centers, I noticed that there were a number of young kinesiologists working under the direction of the physiotherapist, who were involved in organized sports and games with the residents.

The physiotherapy department was not large, but contained the usual type of equipment such as wall bars, weights and pulleys, treatment tables, tumbling mats and a stationery bicycle. The physiotherapist, Isme Roth-Meyer, was a tall slim woman in her early fifties, a halo of braided brown hair around her head and wearing a British tweed suit. One resident, sitting in a wheelchair, was talking to a young man at the far end of the room. It was about ten o'clock in the morning.

"Do sit down," Isme said, in a strong British accent. "Cup of tea ?"

"No thank you Isme," I said. "I just thought it was time we met. I've always worked closely with physiotherapists. We tend to complement each other in so many areas."

"No one works closely with anyone here, you will soon discover, my dear. But I'm pleased to meet you nevertheless. Your project is getting a lot of attention, but then, you must understand, we have no time at all to work with the blind. We're much too busy and short-staffed as it is, and the blind are not good candidates for the games."

"Do you think an exercise program could be arranged for the blind residents in the gym, Isme?" I asked. "They're all young, many are able-bodied, and none of them get enough exercise."

"Most unlikely!" replied Isme. "Our staff have no training for that sort of thing you must understand. We'd like to help, of course, but if they are totally blind they can't see the equipment now, can they? What could they possibly do? I appreciate the interest of the Government in the plight of these people, but really, your program is limited in how far it will go. No one ever goes away from here. It is their home, you see? Where would they go?

You wouldn't want to make them dissatisfied with their lot now, would you? When you've been here a little longer you will learn the philosophy. Do you know the saying, "Be content to accept the things you cannot change?"

"Yes, but I've also heard the rest of it - to change what you can change."

"Not here, my dear. The old ways are always the best. Change is not a good thing here. It just disrupts everything. You won't last, you know, I can tell you that now. No one with new ideas ever lasts here. We can't even keep another physiotherapist. They never stay. But thank you for coming. Nice meeting you."

"May I ask one favour, Isme? I understand that the gym activities are under your direction. May I make use of the gym for my residents?"

"If you insist, of course. Speak to Tom. There may be some spare time. But don't expect any of my staff to run your program."

"But couldn't they help, if I get it started? Surely the blind residents are entitled to use the facilities of the Centre too."

"You are very persistent, aren't you? Are you behind this riding program too, that Dr. Ambrose is talking about? An utterly senseless idea and very dangerous too. That type of program is not suitable at all for blind people and Canadians know nothing whatever about it. Successful in England of course, but impossible here."

I noticed that the gymnasium was completely empty as I walked by.

I had worked in other institutions, and knew that each one was different and took a period of adjustment, but I had a strange feeling that there was an insidious undertow in this place that eventually, inevitably, dragged everyone who stayed beyond a certain period of time down to a level of inertia, where tradition, acceptance of the status quo and an unquestioning process of blind obedience took precedence over reason and initiative. Government communiqués were posted from time to time proclaiming the rights and privileges of the residents, but they were never read or interpreted to the residents. In actual practice there was an almost agnostic disregard for these rights, as though the people for whom they were intended were in some way sub-human or a different species from everyone else.

I decided that reinforcement for the staff was the pay cheque and the security of a government-paid job. In fact, I felt that the staff were as much victims of the system as the residents, because most of them were trapped in the job. If they did not follow the rules, they risked demotion or lack of respect among their peers. Few were trained for any other type of employment. The absentee rate was high, and everyone took full advantage of time off the job because no one was ever actually fired, even after severe reprimand.

But some staff did have different motives for working here, particularly the professional staff who could have found employment elsewhere. Some were truly dedicated, and their reward was not the pay cheque. They were here to serve the most helpless of earth's creatures, because their need was so great. There were probably a few who found an escape here from more demanding responsibilities and some who were new Canadians who had not yet been able to qualify in their professions in Canada, due to a new language or lack of internship opportunities. I stopped along the corridor to look out at the bleak landscape. The leaves had fallen and the trees stood black and bare against the grey sky.

"You look down in the dumps today Sally." It was Philip Martin. "Is the system finally getting to you?"

"Oh Philip, I am glad to see you. Have you time for a cup of coffee? I need to talk to someone."

Chapter 15

DROWNING IN PAPERWORK

"Easy to say somewhere, not so easy to say where."
Charles Dickens

In mid-November, a rehabilitation counselor telephoned me from the city.

"I wonder if you could help me," he said. "My name is John Carlos. I'm calling on behalf of a client named Rikki Chase. We've received conflicting reports about her rehabilitation potential. Your reports appear to give a different impression than the Maplegrove Skills Program, and because Rikki has applied to a group home in this city it's important for us to resolve this problem. Do you think I could meet with you and the others concerned with Rikki some day next week?"

Mr. Carlos explained that my reports indicated a good potential for admission to a group home, whereas the other reports described her as being manipulative, demanding, uneducable, and totally unsuitable for rehabilitation.

I was surprised and angry. I explained that Rikki was indeed manipulative and demanding, but that this was a sign of ability and intelligence, as well as frustration with her present situation, not the opposite, and that while physically she would not be able to walk or perform certain skills, intellectually she had a good potential for rehabilitation in a group home.

Mr. Carlos replied that he did not understand and would have to come for a conference.

I went immediately to see Marianne Gold, who was in charge of the Community Skills program. At my request she drew Rikki's file from the cabinet. "Yes, here it is," she said. "A very low score. No potential at all. Do you know this resident?"

"Yes, indeed I do," I said, defensively. "May I see your test scores?"

I looked over the sheets of tests. "Why this is all motor activity," I exclaimed, "washing dishes, making beds, dressing, getting in and out of a bath tub, reading, handling money, climbing stairs, and of course the inevitable shoe laces."

"Are you saying that she *can* do these things?" asked Marianne.

"Of course not," I replied vehemently. "These are all activities for sighted people who can walk. Rikki has cerebral palsy and is totally blind."

"Then I really don't see how you think she can manage independently in the community," observed Marianne. "She's certainly not a candidate for our program."

"But, don't you see, Marianne? She *could* manage in a group home. She has a good mind. How do you think a quadriplegic manages in a group home?"

"With blindness too? Intellect alone, is not much use with so much disability. What would she do all day? Sit in a corner and be waited on? I'm sorry, but we can't help."

"Would you at least attend a case conference with the rehab officer, Mr. Carlos?"

"Yes, of course Sally, but we would have to report on our own test results."

"Yes," I replied. "And I on mine."

The conference did not go well. In addition to John Carlos from Rehabilitation Services, it was attended by two of Rikki's ward counselors, Marianne Gold from Community Skills, Philip Martin from Social Work, Malcolm O'Shea from Psychology, who had never met Rikki, and me.

"We actually have no proof except your word that Rikki has normal intelligence," John Carlos was saying. "Her behavior on the ward does not seem to indicate it, and without some motor skills and with total blindness, rehabilitation into the community looks somewhat dim. Could we have a psychology test done, Malcolm? The psych test from rehab was not particularly revealing."

"We don't do testing unless the resident is actually being discharged." said Malcolm. "And besides, we have no tests for the blind, so I doubt if the results would be very useful."

"I understand that Rikki has already been refused by the group home," said John. "Did they give any specific reason for their refusal, Sally?"

"Yes. The reason they gave *her* was that she had to be more independent, but the reason they gave *me*, when I called them was that they had a great many applications from people who literally had no place to go, and Rikki actually had a placement here, albeit unsuitable. I find this impossible to accept, because Rikki and both her parents attended the first planning meeting, held at Rehab., for that home, and you will find it in the minutes where they were promised unequivocally that she would be one of the first two residents, because it was unanimously agreed that this institution was the wrong placement for her. In fact, neither of those first two candidates were accepted. The other was Peter Rondo, a young quadriplegic."

"We have re-applied, of course," said Philip. "I suspect that it's the blindness that worries them, because they look at a diagnosis like that, and quadriplegia too, as "heavy care". Initially, until the staff is trained, they're looking for "easy care" residents. We realize that Owen House is not intended to be a home for blind people, just physically disabled, but Rikki should be eligible because she will never be eligible for the Agency for the Blind. What more could we do here, to show that she would be able to manage in that home?"

"I agree with you Philip, about blindness being a major problem," I said. "Everyone's afraid of that. But I think the group home committee are more afraid of mental retardation, and I suspect that's the real stumbling block. This home isn't designed for the mentally retarded. I know that this girl is not retarded, but how can I convince them if I can't even convince you people who work with her?"

"You're the only one who can do that Sally," said John, "because what I'm seeing here is a conflict among all of you who are caring for her. I don't know who to believe."

"Give me three months, John. I'll come up with proof somehow."

I walked back towards my department with Philip. "I know how discouraged you must feel Sally," he said, "after all your work with Rikki. We're going to have to do something different to convince them."

"Yes. I know. I'm going to telephone the Department of Education tomorrow. Maybe they would send us a correspondence course. I've got to prove to someone that she has learning ability. Any other ideas?"

"There's one possibility, Sally. I'm going to call Palmer House in Stemler. You said they were approached before when Rikki was at Rehab. I'll explain the problem and maybe they'll take her this time just for a trial period. After all, that home was specially designed for young people with cerebral palsy and if she did well there, it might help us to get her in somewhere else. I'll explain how important this is for her."

"It's certainly worth a try, Philip. Do you think her parents would let her go?"

"We've kept in touch with them all along, Sally. I don't see why they would object. Let's give it a try. I'll call you as soon as I have an answer. And go ahead and look into the correspondence idea. What subject would you choose? English? History?"

"No. She doesn't have the vocabulary or the comprehension for that yet. I was thinking of Grade 9 French. It's basic and mainly depends on memory and very basic grammar, and it's something she has never learned. It needs to be something totally new to her, to prove our point."

Philip took the stairway up to his office as I continued along the corridor, thinking of what I would say to the Ministry of Education.

A few days later, two counselors from the Agency for the Blind came to visit the ward, Mr. Carter and Mrs. Dodds. Both were legally blind. They spent an hour on the ward meeting the residents and staff and then I took them to lunch in the staff dining room.

"Of course we would like to help you Sally," said Mr. Carter, "but it will be at least five months before we can let you have a brailler."

"It's not a brailler we need right now," I said. "Rikki was tested at Rehab for learning Braille, but because of impaired tactile discrimination in her fingers, and the use of only one hand, she was unable to learn Braille. We need "Talking Book" machines and tapes. Why is it so difficult to get them? I understand that the Agency audio tapes can't be played on other tape players, so we have to get a player through you, in order to use your Talking Books."

"They're very expensive and we only have a certain allotment for the region. I'll see what I can do, but I can't promise anything in the near future. We'll try to send a field worker out as soon as possible, but we're short there too, because our man who used to cover this region has been transferred to another area. The first step, of course, is to register everyone."

"But Mr. Carter, most of our residents have been registered since birth. Doesn't that entitle them to at least some services from the Agency?"

"It's a long way out here from the city," said Mr. Carter. "We're always very short of workers for regions out of the city."

My request for a correspondence course for Rikki was relayed through the Department of Education to a secretary who telephoned to ask why a grade nine course had been requested for someone who had never had any previous education. I explained the purpose of the course, that Rikki was an adult, and in order to maintain interest it had to have some content on a higher level than Dick and Jane. I explained that I would be supervising the course myself and that I felt the content should be at an adult level, but at the same time very basic.

The secretary sounded dubious because they had never had a similar request, but with the promise of professional supervision, she agreed to send the material on trial. A package of books, pre-addressed envelopes and the first three assignments arrived in the mail the following week. Then I was faced with the problem of finding a quiet place for Rikki to begin her French studies, as well as to continue with her reading.

Marigold Brown had been the secretary in occupational therapy for many years. She had a friendly manner with the residents and a pleasant telephone voice so that her social skills made up for any shortcomings she might have had in typing and spelling. Marigold enjoyed her job as long as it did not make any unpredictable demands. She liked routine. She agreed to allow Rikki to work in the department under her surveillance, as long as she was not required to make decisions or show any initiative.

I would plan all the assignments, and this would assure that Rikki was off the ward for most of every day. In off hours, I recorded radio programs, stories from other tapes, short lessons in French, and questions on the reading, with music to fill the gaps. Rikki was encouraged to spend several hours on one tape if necessary, and to learn its contents. Her answers to the questions would indicate how well she understood each story before going on to the next. At most, I was spending about half an hour a day with Rikki, and for this reason I was taken completely by surprise when I received a memo from Dr. Ambrose, advising me to reduce my input into Rikki's program. I went immediately to Dr. Ambrose's office.

"I appreciate your interest in this case, Sally," Dr. Ambrose was saying, in his usual hesitant way, "but it appears that there have been objections... complaints that you are spending too much time with Rikki at the expense of the other residents."

"Too much time, Dr. Ambrose? This was incredulous. Who is making these complaints? Do they know exactly how much time I spend with Rikki, and with the others? Are they aware that I prepare all of Rikki's lessons in the evening in my own time?"

"I can't really give you the source of the complaints, Sally, but Mr. Nash has asked me to convey to you that you might spend less time with this particular resident, if it is causing a conflict."

I was utterly dumfounded. I could hardly believe it. I knew that Dr. Ambrose approved of what I was doing, and I suspected that he had been given this unpleasant assignment against his own judgment. I lacked a ready reply, struggling to keep my emotions in check.

Then: "Dr. Ambrose, I've always kept you informed about what we're doing with the blind residents. You know that the program has been a huge success so far. You also know that Rikki has a good chance of getting out of here into the real world, and that she won't get out unless we can prove that she has a potential. That's what I'm trying to do. All my preparation for Rikki is done after hours, in my own time, with my own tapes. Rikki is blossoming under the program. Anyone can see that. Why does the staff want everyone here to be functioning on the same low level?"

Dr. Ambrose looked out the window and after a moment replied in a lower voice, "Tell me, Sally, how many others, in your opinion, should not be here?"

I thought for a minute. "I think there are many who should not be here, but perhaps I could say that there are a great many who should not have come in the first place. They've been taught to be retarded, and they're being kept that way. Just look at what's happening on the blind ward. None of them are ready to go out yet, because there is no suitable place for people who are that dependent, and they haven't got the social skills yet to manage in the real world, but they will be able to, eventually, if the program works. Right now, Rikki, and perhaps Peer, are the closest to making it. That's why I can't stop now with Rikki."

"Right," replied Dr. Ambrose, looking uncomfortable. "Well, let's just say that I told you." He rose from his desk and walked with me to the door.

I wandered slowly down the hall. I was not angry any more. Dr. Ambrose was a sad, gentle, unassertive man, caught in the system, like everyone else on this satellite so removed from reality. So they were warning me to stop working with Rikki. Well, I'll show them how that tactic will work, I thought. I was now determined to strive even harder with Rikki and leave no stone unturned to get her out of this "prison" as soon as possible.

The inter-facility conference was planned for mid-January. By mid-December there was a full complement of eighteen residents on the ward, the dining room furniture was a successful addition, volunteers from a local community college had been found to help out on the ward once a week, and staff morale was the highest it had ever been.

Everything was going ahead except the riding program. Funding had still not been approved, and Dr. Ambrose, while still sounding optimistic, was evasive about details.

One day. I was asked to meet with Claire in the O.T. department. She placed two cups of coffee on the desk and lit a cigarette. I always tried to meet with Claire at least once a week, but she still had little understanding, or interest in my work and seldom asked any serious questions about it.

Claire was a good O.T., but had been involved in administrative work for many years and was now close to retirement. She liked to trust her therapists to manage their own affairs, as long as they touched base with her regularly and the reports came in on time. I had submitted reports regularly, but I suspected that Claire filed most of them without reading them. But I enjoyed talking to her.

She was a good listener and tended to bring out the best in people. I had told her about my frustrations with the constant delays in the riding program.

"I've found out why your riding program has been held up, Sally," she was saying. "I should have realized that it would have to be approved by the P.A.C.".

"Whatever is the P.A.C.?"

"The Professional Advisory Council. All programs have to be presented in a special format. I have a copy here. You have to write out all the details according to a Government directive..."

She passed a copy to me. There were headings, such as "Committee", "Purpose of Program", "Results and Method of Measurement", "Is Program Desirable?", "Is Program Measurable?", "Is Program Attainable?", "Is it specific?", "Is it End Oriented?", "Short term Goals", "Long Term Goals", "First Objective,", "Second Objective"....

"Oh come on, Claire! Do we really have to do all this? These questions were all answered in my original brief."

"Better get on with it as soon as possible, Sally."

"Do you know how much time I spend on paperwork already, Claire?"

"Yes, we all do, Sally, but it's important to do this right away because the next P.A.C. conference will be next week, and there won't be another for at least a month. You'll have to attend the conference and defend your report if it is accepted."

My proposal was accepted by the P.A.C. and I was instructed to present myself at the board room at three o'clock the following Wednesday afternoon.

Twelve people sat around the long oak table. At first glance I did not recognize anyone. Then I noticed that Marianne Gold was acting Chairman in place of Mr.

Nash, an equally discouraging alternative. A tray with a glass jug of ice water and tumblers occupied a spot in the centre of the table. Each person had copies of several briefs with mine on top. I suddenly felt on trial. Nobody smiled.

After I had taken my place in the only vacant chair, Marianne introduced the members of the Committee around the table. I recognized a few names, for the most part they were social workers, psychologists, and some senior personnel and counselor staff. I wondered what any of them knew about riding programs.

"We have all read your submission, Sally," said Marianne. "Now we have a few questions. We will start on my left."

One by one, each person asked a question. No similar program had ever been suggested and they were concerned about the safety elements and about the advisability of having a program taking place beyond the grounds of the institution. None of them had ever worked with the blind or visited the ward and no one had even gone over to look at the stable.

"I'm concerned about the cost," said one committee member. "Five dollars a week per resident seems excessive, compared with other programs that don't cost anything."

"The cost is actually extremely reasonable," I explained. "You must understand that we're paying for animals that have had to be trained, fed and cared for, saddled up and un-tacked each time, as well as the expertise of the instructor and the use of the arena. The regular cost of lessons at any stable is at least three times this much. They've given us a special price."

"Where do you intend to get volunteers to help you during the day-time hours?" asked another.

"The local high school has offered to send students if we'll provide the transportation," I replied. "At first we'll need helpers to lead the horses as well as side-walkers for each horse. The high school is very interested in this program and wants to help. They think it would be a good experience for their students."

"There's another expense," said the previous speaker. "We're not here to help the high school."

"I think the benefits of the program will outweigh any costs," I said.

By four o'clock the committee was still arguing about transportation, safety, clothing, equipment, until I despaired that the program would ever get off the ground. I could hardly believe my ears when one committee member, a psychologist, stated, "I don't see why dogs wouldn't do just as well and be a hell of a lot cheaper."

No one laughed. He was serious. I was so appalled at his complete misunderstanding of all that had preceded that I lacked a ready answer and gave no reply.

I was told that I could leave and that I would be informed of the results in due time. It had been a long day.

Slowly, I began the long walk down to the other end of "Main Street", feeling completely deflated. I wondered if it was all worth it. I could get a much nicer job in the city. Today escape seemed more desirable than ever. None of these people cared one bit about the residents. All they cared about was their own egos and their predictable pay cheques, safely predictable as long as they spouted the party line, kept their noses clean, did not rock the boat, and didn't loose the "merchandise" because, to them, the residents were no more than commodities. By the time I had reached the crossroads of the next corridor I was reacting with anger and discouragement.

"Hi Sally. How did it go?" How was it that Philip always seemed to turn up at such opportune moments?

"Terrible! It was simply awful. How does that lot ever make a decision about anything? The problem really is, Philip, that none of them know anything about blindness, or about what we've been doing. I can't understand why psychologists would not have more insight, because I know they're qualified psychologists, but even doctors don't understand the implication of a severe visual handicap, or they would never have signed many of these people into the institution in the first place."

"That's right, Sally, I suspect it has something to do with labeling people, and our people can't be labeled because they all have several disabilities and don't fit any one, and one disability exaggerates the other. Let's go and get a cup of coffee. You look drained."

"Yes, I am," I said, as we walked slowly towards the coffee shop. "How do you think health professionals can become so narrow, so specialized that they can't see the whole person any more? They all seem to put controls on how far they will go to help a patient, and this isn't because they're avoiding treading on someone else's territory. It seems more because they don't want to put enough effort into problem solving. Our clients are disabled adult citizens of this country, yet they don't have any appropriate treatment services. Isn't that terrible?"

"It's discouraging, Sally, but cheer up. You'll get your program. I heard that your proposal was the best they've ever had."

Chapter 16

IF YOU COULD SEE WHAT I HEAR

"Listening to a tale being told in the dark is one of the most ancient of man's entertainments."
Moss Hart

After my last meeting with Dr Ambrose, I decided that I would have to increase the time I spent with Rikki to try to get faster results, in case I was forced to discontinue her lessons during the day. This would, of course, have to be done in my own time. I decided to work with her one evening a week.

The following Wednesday evening I had dinner in the staff dining room and then picked up Rikki on the ward. There was no objection from the staff and she was delighted to be going out. I decided to use my own office on the third floor for these sessions.

We would have to use the freight elevator at the north end of the building. This gave me an opportunity to teach Rikki how to estimate distances. I attached a wooden clothes pin to one wheel of her chair, so that it made a click sound with each revolution of the wheel. By counting clicks, she could compare distances. The main corridor, usually so busy and noisy, was almost deserted at this time. Shadows loomed in the alcoves and doorways that led out to the grounds. The sound of my footsteps and the clicking of the clothes pin echoed from the walls. As we approached the elevator a solitary cleaner was scrubbing window sills and baseboards along the corridor.

Rikki kept up an incessant chatter along the way. "This reminds me of the time Chrissie and I were lost," she was saying. "Chrissie offered to take me for a walk, but we went the wrong way, and we walked and walked and didn't know where we were. After awhile I called out to people going past. Chrissie didn't want to say anything but I'm not shy, and I kept asking people to help us, and you know what happened? Nobody would answer. They just kept walking by."

"That must have been very frightening, Rikki," I said. "What did you do then?"

"Well, after a long time - about an hour I guess, I had to go… you know… to the toilet, so I started to cry. And then, thank God, Reverent Jones came by, and he knew us and took us back. It was scary."

I was hoping I would be able to operate the freight elevator, because I had never used it before. As a rule we never took residents upstairs to the therapy offices, but the elevator presented no problem and there would be no one else there in the evening. We emerged from the elevator in almost complete darkness, too early for moonlight. I found a light switch and drew up a chair opposite Rikki at a small table. We had been reading an autobiography by Tom Sullivan, called "If You Could See What I Hear", about his experience as a young blind student attending the Perkins boarding school for the blind in the United States.

This book had given me an insight into the sort of problems blind people had in the real world, and I thought Rikki could relate to it. We had reached the part where the writer was describing his experience when he attended his first dance. This held her full attention. Tom had never realized that women were physically different from men. Back in the residence after the party Tom was describing to his room mate his excitement when he held his partner close in his arms.

His room mate expressed concern that Tom had held her so close. "You might have gotten her pregnant!" he declared. Tom was so appalled that he went to his priest, who burst out laughing. So did I. Suddenly Rikki hit the table with her fist. "What's funny?" she asked in a loud voice.

Up to this time Rikki had expressed no interest in the opposite sex, apart from her questions about animals and, like the other blind residents, she had never been taught anything about sexuality or gender differences between male and female. The story about Tom's experiences not only awakened an interest for more information, but dispelled a number of misconceptions that Rikki had picked up on the ward. I answered as clearly and simply as possible, as one would to a child, because she tended to turn off if the discussion got too detailed. She wanted to know how people got pregnant, where babies came from, and why there was so much concern when one of the girls got pregnant on the ward.

The more I read to Rikki the more I realized that I could reach her innate intelligence and understanding through stories. She had never been aware of other people's problems. Her whole world had been centered within herself. Conversation on the ward, if it was intelligible at all, was limited to basic bodily functions, and it was not considered proper for staff to talk about their personal life to residents. Residents were accustomed to having all decisions made for them. They had no opportunity to decide what to wear, what to eat, where to go, when to go to bed, when to get up, and as a result they had no experience with problem solving, were never allowed to make a mistake.

I was just beginning to think about taking Rikki back to the ward when suddenly the power went off and we were in total darkness. "Oh - oh!", I said.

"What's the matter Sally?"

I explained that the lights had gone out and we would have to wait awhile until they came on again.

"But you have to go home. Well, you don't have to worry, I can tell you where to go. It's all the same to me, and you taught me the way. I know how far we have to go because I counted the clicks on the wheel."

"Good for you. And now the tables are reversed, except for one problem, Rikki. The elevator won't work without power, and I don't want to take you down the stairs in your wheelchair. I could go and get help, but I don't want to leave you here alone either. I'll see if I can find the telephone."

"Maybe we'll be stuck here too late for you to go home. I could arrange for you to sleep with me on the ward."

I was surprised at my reaction to this generous suggestion, to sleep with Rikki in her narrow little iron cot with the thin cotton sheet over the cold rubber-covered mattress. It was a purely generous offer from Rikki, but the suggestion filled me with nothing short of revulsion, followed by shame, that this could be acceptable for Rikki and not for me.

As I tried to remember exactly how far away the stairs were, in case I had to go and get help, and then try to find the telephone to call the ward, I realized that I would have to do this exactly as a blind person would. This was considerably different from wearing a blindfold that could be taken off.

I groped my way across the room. Not being a smoker, I didn't even have a cigarette lighter. Distances seemed quite different in the dark and I walked into some furniture before finding my desk. I dialed "O" for the switchboard and was relieved when I got an answer and thankful that I didn't have to dial a full number, because I had no way of looking it up in the directory, and I had not taught myself the method blind people use to dial a telephone. I was amazed at how inept I was. I asked the operator to send help if the lights didn't come on soon, and to tell someone on Rikki's ward that if the power did come on I would have to trust it not to go off again while we were still in the elevator. If this should happen, we could be there all night.

After about ten minutes the lights came on, to my great relief, and I was able to take Rikki back to the ward. I wondered how long we might have been trapped in the elevator, because the night staff would not expect anyone to be using it in the evening. Yet it was unlikely that Rikki would not have been missed before bedtime.

So often I was aware that I was continually learning along with Rikki, and this was very largely because I was spending enough time with her. I had now recorded six books, and I was beginning to notice, a slow but steady improvement in Rikki's use of language and ability to ask questions, as well as comprehension.

I was becoming increasingly aware of the importance of language for blind people, and I realized now that regular "Talking Books" would be too difficult for Rikki without some explanation as the story developed, because she still tended to turn off if she did not understand a passage. I thought of the anecdote about three blind men and an elephant, each one feeling a different part of the animal and concluding that an elephant was like a wall, or a tree trunk, or a rope. If we had been able to get the "Talking Books" earlier, Rikki might never have learned to really listen to stories.

Sighted people often read about something they have never seen, but understand it from a clear description, or even better, from a picture. It has been said that a picture is worth a thousand words. Therefore, by the same token, a blind person would need a thousand words to fully understand one picture. No wonder it takes more time for a blind person to learn, particularly if he or she has been blind from birth like Rikki.

Through words I was hoping to open a new world for Rikki, a world of new things, new experiences, and a way of learning how people deal with events that affect their lives. How else could she learn normal behavior, how to react normally to adverse situations, and gradually to have some control over her own life? At the same time, I was introducing Rikki to more and more music. She seemed to enjoy listening to it and it saved me some reading time in between stories. I recorded some of the more popular classics, such as Chopin and Strauss waltzes, ballet and marching music, different types of instrumental music and singing. I knew that she had extraordinary hearing, and could recognize sounds and voices much better than I could. I now realized that Rikki had a good ear for music.

The next day I met with Douglas Prior, Director of Volunteers, to review the transportation issues and costs for the riding program proposal. Doug's office was on the second floor in another part of the building - an area used exclusively for office management. In an institution of this size the Director of Volunteers had a busy and responsible full-time job, because volunteers provided many necessary services and had to be carefully screened and supervised.

Doug mentioned that his Secretary, Mary Smith, would be away next week for two weeks. This presented a problem, because he had not been able to find a replacement, and there were no answering machines at this time. I decided to suggest an idea. I asked if he would consider allowing a resident to answer the telephone and take messages for him. I was thinking of Rikki. She had a strong clear voice, she knew how to put the messages on her tape recorder, and this would give her another opportunity to show that she could learn work skills. It would be part of her treatment program.

Douglas Prior was a kind man and accustomed to a great variety of people helping out at the institution. He said he would give Rikki a try. I agreed to help her get started and would bring her up the next day while the secretary was still there. Rikki was thrilled at being given a real job to do and took to the telephone duties with no problems whatsoever. It freed Doug from answering a very busy telephone, allowing him to return the calls in his own time, and he expressed total satisfaction with the arrangement.

I was therefore surprised when I was summoned to a meeting with the secretarial pool across the hall from Doug's office. The senior secretary was furious about the arrangement. She explained to me in a loud voice that carried right across the hall to Rikki, that residents were not allowed on this floor. This was *staff territory*, and Rikki would have to go.

When I met with Doug about this, in his usual quiet way he told me not to worry about it. He had employed Rikki and that was the end of it.

My life continued to be full of surprises. The following week I was again summoned to the same office, and was not looking forward to another confrontation. To my surprise, in the presence of all her staff, the secretary apologized to me for her complaint, and said that they were all amazed at the excellent job that Rikki was doing. They had all decided that she could stay.

Chapter17

MOVING FORWARD

"There is something about the outside of a horse that is good for the inside of a man."
Liam O'Flaherty

As winter set in activities on the ward had increased to include games designed to teach skills such as finding their way independently around the ward, the wash room and the bedroom areas as well as basic table manners. We were now allowed to use a shower room down the hall for bathing, instead of the hated hose and slab, and residents had learned to comb their own hair and brush their teeth. The tooth brushes had all been marked or placed in a certain way so that each resident could recognize his or her own. Eating had become a pleasure, particularly when they learned the names of the food they were eating and the competition to grab and eat fast was no longer necessary. And there was no problem with misuse of toilet paper.

But something more exciting was happening. The newly learned freedom of movement and expression was promoting a happy social interaction that the residents had never experienced before. Personalities began to develop as well as friendships. They were becoming like a family. They knew that the staff liked them and they liked and trusted us, and they knew that we cared about what they did and what they thought. This was leading to bonding, something that had previously been discouraged, because formerly, when a resident became too fond of a certain member of staff, that employee was moved to another ward. There were no false goals. The reward was a new achievement resulting from a new challenge.

Christmas brought extra volunteers to the institution to relieve the staff shortage over the holiday season. The wards on the unit decided to have a competition to see which ward had the best decorations. Special B was no exception, and although most of the residents could not see the bright colours and designs, they knew they were there and saw them through the eyes of the others. The spirit of the festive season was received with joy and excitement by everyone, and the residents were more aware than they had ever been of what was going on.

Santa and his entourage trooped onto the ward on the twenty-third of December, the day designated as Christmas. We were all seated around a large artificial tree surrounded by presents, waiting for Santa to distribute the gifts. I wondered what the blind residents thought of this custom, particularly when the tree had no natural fiber and no scent, and looked, and felt, for all the world like a tall pole with large bottle brushes for branches.

The traditional presents, the necessities for next year, such as socks, pajamas, underwear, shaving cream and tooth paste, were unwrapped by each person in turn, the staff making appropriate sounds of admiration. Then Santa began to distribute a special present to each person, something unknown in previous years. These were donated by interested benefactors who wanted to help the special ward. Chrissie was given a guitar that would have been soon broken on any other ward. Harry got a pocket radio. He did not understand immediately what it was because it had no batteries, but he was pleased. A few days later I took Harry to a radio shop in the town and showed him how to buy the batteries he needed to make the radio work. His pleasure showed no bounds.

Peer was delighted with his new padlock, to lock his box under his bed, with his own key. Ten residents received Braille watches. But Tony received the most exciting gift of all, an electric organ the size of a small piano. He commenced to play it immediately with sheer and utter delight. Tony had learned to play hymns that he had heard in chapel on the old piano that I had promoted for the ward and therefore was able to learn to play the organ immediately.

It was a sad reflection on society that most small gifts usually disappeared shortly after Christmas, but this was unlikely to happen on this ward. The watches, records and other valuables were carefully put away, waiting for training in how to use them.

Harry's pocket radio stayed safely inside his shirt - his first and most prized personal possession. Rory's little harmonica unfortunately fell apart and was lost when he removed the screws, but Chrissie's guitar did not meet the predicted fate. He stroked the strings so lovingly that Bob, the chaplain's assistant, took an interest in teaching him, and Chrissie responded with unexpected aptitude. As Chrissie repeated the exercises Bob had given him he gradually began to play recognizable tunes.

* * *

Christmas was hardly over before Dr. Piercey, Mikaela, paid another visit to set the framework for the

Inter-Institutional Conference, to be held in two weeks. Each senior staff member had been given the responsibility of presenting a paper on one aspect of the ward program. Mikaela explained the importance for staff from all the institutions to be given an opportunity to share ideas, learn together and establish relationships partly because they were all good people, but also because they were all pioneers, working in isolation. While I felt that everything was happening much too fast, I decided that any shortcomings could be blamed on the newness of the program.

On the day of the conference, visitors entered the ward in small groups. The residents were wearing their best clothes and looked remarkably normal. I listened with interest to the comments of the visitors: "Listen! They're actually talking to each other!"... "Hey, look! They're allowed to have possessions! Look at that guitar. And he even plays it!"... "The ward is so clean! The bathroom doesn't even smell!"

Several people from the Government attended too, which pleased me. The papers were received with interest and it was decided to make the conference an annual event. Mikaela was pleased too, and congratulated us on the results, although I had the feeling that she had expected no less. Everyone was relieved that it had been such a success.

The riding program was finally approved in February and ten residents were selected who could tolerate the cold weather. The weekly classes were to be conducted according to the accepted format of a riding school as closely as possible. Our instructor was qualified to teach disabled riders and the horses were quiet, well trained and obedient. My role, as "therapist on the ground", was to watch for fatigue or other problems as well as suggesting any necessary adaptations. Additional time was allowed for riders to explore the stable and learn about stable management, feeding and grooming. High school volunteers and one or two ward staff were taught to lead the horses and act as side-walkers.

Initially six residents; Harry, Chrissie, Donny, Rory, Colin and Tony made up the first group of riders. As I helped them with their coats and boots, I wondered if any of them had any idea of what a horse was really like. To them, this was an outing in a van, and that was sufficient cause for excitement. They did not expect to understand anything beyond that.

On the way to the stable I explained to them that a stable was a house for horses. When we arrived the student volunteers were already tacking up the horses, cross-tied in the aisle. I assigned two students to each resident, and after being allowed to feel the horses, saddles and bridles, all proceeded to the arena that was attached to the stable.

When Tony suddenly realized that he would actually be sitting on the horse's back he expressed misgivings about the animal's ability to hold him. Rory wanted to know where the horses went to the bathroom, and this in turn gave Colin the idea that he had to go, so a student was dispatched to take him up to the farm house.

I broke off an icicle hanging in the stable doorway for the riders to feel, then noticed that Colin was whimpering and shaking his hands. "My hands hurt," he said, "and something keeps touching my face." Then I realized that Colin had never felt cold or falling snow before.

The success of the riding program was astounding. The security of the astride position in the saddle along with the even cadence of the horse in the walk and trot, resulted in improved walking in the ward and the gym, something these residents had never experienced. We also noticed improvement in expressive language, muscle tone and more awareness of the environment. Gradually, more riders were added to the program and a second class was started.

One day, an exciting thing happened. Benny, a boy who had been diagnosed with Down's Syndrome as well as total congenital blindness, and had always been completely non-verbal, was seated on a horse. He was obviously very excited by the experience. The instructor walked over to Benny and asked him if he liked riding the horse. Very slowly Benny replied, "Y-e-s... I... do." Then she asked, "Are you coming again next week?" and Benny replied, "Y-e-s... I am." These were the first words Benny had ever spoken. I was most excited about Benny's sudden ability to talk, because I had read that the vestibular system, concerned with equilibrium and our ability to adjust to gravity, is related to the speech mechanism, but I had never seen it happen before.

Molly came with the second group. She had not been included originally, partly because of her loud voice that might frighten the horses, but also because she was hemiplegic with a left side paralysis, and would require more experienced helpers to assure that she would not loose her balance and fall off.

As expected, Molly did lean to one side, presenting a problem for the side walker who was having some difficulty supporting her in an upright position. I suggested that the student who was leading the horse should walk forward at a more even working pace, while the side walker merely put her hand firmly on Molly's thigh. As I expected, as the horse moved on, Molly straightened herself up and found her own balance.

The riding program introduced new concepts, but also new situations that these young people had never experienced before. One day before the riding class started I introduced Chrissie to one of the sheep that had wandered over, near the stable. Chrissie was excited by the woolly feel and the size and shape of the sheep. He had never felt any animals before.

Seeing his excitement, Peter, one of the helpers, brought a large hen over and placed it in Chrissie's arms. Feeling the feathers, Chrissie exclaimed, "What is *this*?"

"It's a hen, Chrissie, a chicken, a kind of bird," he said. " These are feathers. All birds have feathers."

"But what's it *for*? What does it *do*?"

"It lays eggs, Chrissie. You know… the kind of eggs you have for breakfast?"

"No kidding!" he exclaimed. "You mean it lays scrambled eggs ?"

Blind and visually impaired people can do well in equestrian programs. Only 10% of legally blind people are totally blind, so if they have only minimal vision they can locate themselves quite well in an arena by the light from the windows. After about a year in the program, most of our riders had learned to trot over cavaletti, two had fallen off their horses without injury and were able to laugh about it, and one boy, Charlie learned to canter on a lunge line while we were filming the program. It was an exciting moment when he, a previously non-verbal rider, called out, "I've got it! I've got it!"

But incredible difficulties persisted. A resident who had been encouraged to anticipate the riding experience every week would be sent to the barber or the dentist on riding days, and another resident would be sent in his place, who had not been screened for the program. In addition to my own screening tests, I was careful to have signed medical approval for each resident, to assure that he or she had no condition that would be adversely affected by the program, such as severe allergies, back or hip problems, or cardiac involvement. Every week some residents would arrive improperly dressed, with sneakers instead of boots with heels, mitts instead of gloves, or the van would be diverted somewhere else the morning of the class.

Sometimes, I had to borrow a vehicle from the city to be sure of transportation so that the class would not have to be canceled. I felt that continuity in programming was something these residents had never had, and I particularly wanted them to be able to anticipate the riding every week. In the past, outdoor programs were usually canceled in inclement weather and as a result, many of the riders had never been outdoors in the rain, snow or cold.

The high school volunteers had been selected by the principal from a group of students who were not doing well in school, in the hope that a program like this might motivate them. Without exception they responded with enthusiasm, initially because it gave them some time away from school, but it was later reported that their studies improved as a result.

One such student named Joan arrived the first day with totally improper clothing for walking in a riding arena, and expressed fear of horses and aversion to all forms of exercise. Initially, she was given the responsibility of side-walker, to be alert to the safety of the rider and re-enforce the commands from the instructor.

As she helped with the program, Joan gradually developed more confidence, and soon she even agreed to have a short ride herself after class. We encouraged the helpers to do this, partly as a reward for helping, but also to teach them what it was like to ride with their eyes closed.

The arena was attached to the stable. Riders, who were able, had been taught to remove the saddles and bridles from their horses and carry them from the arena along the stable hallway to the tack room. This was not only considered good exercise, but the weight and size of the tack helped to re-enforce their impression of the size of the horse. One day, as the riders were carrying their tack from the arena, one of the horses broke loose and bolted for his stall, heading straight for little Donald who was walking along the aisle with his saddle, right in the path of the horse. Responding immediately, Joan, who was nearest to the door, jumped in front of the horse with her arms outstretched, veering the animal back into the arena. I telephoned the principal of the school in praise of this student for her quick thinking, that possibly averted a serious accident. I hoped that this act of courage would lead to success for this girl at school.

* * *

Volunteers from the community were always welcome on the ward, but most required a certain amount of training and supervision. I was careful not to subdue their natural exuberance, but sometimes it conflicted with the methods being used to teach normal behavior.

One day a community college student named Missy bounced onto the ward with such exuberance that I thought she must have known the residents before. Not content with shaking hands, as they were being taught to do as a substitute for eye contact, Missy was hugging and kissing them like long-lost friends. I watched this performance for awhile, then took Missie aside.

"May I make a suggestion, Missy?" I asked. "When you meet someone you don't know on the street in town, what do you do?"

"Why, just say "Hi", I guess."

"You don't hug or kiss them when you first meet them?"

"No."

"Then why do you do that here?"

"Well, I don't know, I thought this was how they act. I was told that the retarded are very affectionate. Aren't they?"

"Yes, that's true, Missy. Some do tend to be overly affectionate. But we're trying to teach them normal behavior. We'd prefer that they learn by your example, and not that you would mimic their behavior."

I was now giving one lesson a week to community college students, as part of my program. Not all the students were keen about working with the blind, but one in particular, named Simon, was keenly interested, and had volunteered to work on one of the other wards where there were a few blind residents. One morning, I was reviewing my program for the day when Simon telephoned. He said that he was calling from a pay telephone, and stressed that this call was strictly confidential.

It transpired that Simon had been working with a deaf-blind girl of about twelve years old. This child usually spent her days curled up on the floor in the corner of the ward. Simon had been teaching her some communication skills and had been making some progress.

The ward Supervisor had summoned Simon to his office and told him in a belligerent manner that he was to stop working with this child. He told Simon that he was wasting his time trying to teach anyone on this ward and he could better occupy himself folding linen. When Simon persisted he was warned that unless he stopped completely, something might happen to him on his way home. I was able to have Simon moved to another ward. I later heard that he had left the institution.

Another day two community college students, who were also working part-time at the institution, asked if they could talk to me privately. Peggy had been crying and Bruce had come with her for support.

"I can't believe what I saw on ward F," Peggy began. "The staff are so cruel."

"In what way are they being cruel?" I asked.

"Well, there's this little guy named Billy," said Peggy, sniffing and reaching for her handkerchief. "He's only about this high... and doesn't know what's going on. One of the staff, Sonya, keeps yelling at him all the time, and today she gave him a big push into a chair. Then this other counselor, Jack, comes out and shouts at Billy to get the hell out of that chair... and you know... they keep doing it."

"Yes," said Bruce, "it's true. I saw it too. It's a kind of game they play. The poor little kid just takes it. We don't want to work on that ward any more. We thought you could do something about it."

This was always a delicate situation, when students would report incidents of cruelty that would be overlooked by staff, because no employee ever wanted to complain. There was always danger of backlash. They preferred silence to rocking the boat.

Incidents like this did not occur often, but when they did they were usually caused by staff burn-out, fatigue, and frustration with the repetitive unrewarding nature of the job.

I had to make a formal complaint to my department head, who, in turn, reported to the unit director, and he to the ward supervisor. I never heard that anything had actually been done except that the students were moved to another ward.

I joined Philip for a cup of coffee that day at four o'clock. I was telling him about the incident on ward F.

This is the problem with institutions," he said. "Even with the best intentions, big institutions always seem to defeat their original purpose. It's a bit like some boarding schools. They tend to bring out the best or the worst in people, particularly if these people have any power."

"Well, they say power corrupts," I said. "but it's also the system. Some staff have been here for over twenty-five years, came when they were sixteen or seventeen, and never had another job or other training. Others come and last two days, or at most, two weeks. It isn't everyone who can stand it."

I helped myself to another cup of coffee, then continued. "It's partly the type of work, the ugliness of it, the smell, the hopelessness, as well as the long hours on your feet, heavy lifting of severely disabled people who can't help, the boring repetition of washing, dressing, feeding - just keeping them alive, and for what purpose?"

Philip did not answer for awhile. Then he said, "There are a lot of contradictions in an institutional setting. There's the misuse of power, usually by people who have never had any, but at the same time the fear of being locked into a system where they have no real control. There's the fear of making a decision and being blamed if it goes wrong. We professionals are the lucky ones because we can easily get a job somewhere else. Most of the ward counselors are not trained for anything else. We don't have to stay, not if the purpose goes. We'll stay as long as we think we're achieving something."

"Do you feel you're achieving something, Philip? Do you like your work?"

Philip laughed. "Yes... and no." Then there was a dreamy look in his eyes. "You know what I'd like? I'd like to close this place and start over... with small homes... everybody else lives in a home, why shouldn't these people? But I guess that's impossible. In the first place, the parents would be against it. They scream like hell if they find some other resident wearing their child's clothes, but they're scared to death of having to look after that child themselves."

Philip paused for a moment, then continued. "Yet… it's not quite right to say that, Sally. I don't blame the parents. They don't know how to look after these people, and they're not getting any younger. What we need is small, well run, group homes, with younger people staffing them, who have the right training, where they can use normal community facilities and where the parents can come to see them and take them out now and then if they like. Families can't cope with them as they are, but where can they go? Do you know what we social workers have been doing? We just shuffle them around. We never really get them into the mainstream."

"Now *you're* getting pessimistic, Philip, and you're my only real ally. You still believe that Rikki can get out, don't you?"

"I hope… I really hope so. But Sally, if we don't place her pretty soon it'll be too late. People are more likely to accept her when she's young. It's getting harder to place the older ones. Are you willing to wait ten years?"

"Oh come on, Philip. I'm going to get Rikki into that home if it's the last thing I do. Not just because I promised Rikki, and not just because I want to prove something. It's because I really believe she can make it. And I'm convinced it won't take ten years. Why doesn't anyone else believe she can do it?"

"I do, Sally. We're still on the same team, right?"

"Philip, sometimes I think you're the only sane person in this place. Well, let's concentrate on getting

Rikki out. Haven't you heard anything yet from Palmer House?"

"Just delays. How's Rikki doing in French?"

"Straight As. Ninety percent, actually. Once she's grasped it she never forgets. She's got an incredible memory. We're up to lesson seven. Well, got to go. Let me know if you hear any *good* news."

Chapter 18

PROGRESS AT LAST

"It is not enough for a man to know how to ride; he must know how to fall."
Mexican Proverb

It was a brisk March day. The wind rattled the windows of the corridor, slammed doors and whistled around the wings of the building. As I walked across the lobby the receptionist called to me, "Oh Sally, Mr. Martin in social work has been trying to reach you."

I turned to the right and went up the stairs to Philip's office.

"Guess what!" Exclaimed Philip. "We have a letter from Palmer House. They've offered to take Rikki for a three week assessment period, starting in mid-April."

"Wow! At last. Now it's going to be up to Rikki. This is just the break we needed."

Philip would make all the arrangements. First he'd contact her parents. If they agreed, he'd write a reply to the letter, then begin the paper work for her temporary release and the required medical tests. I was given the pleasant duty of telling her, which I decided to delay until we were certain that her parents would let her go.

"She'll have to be taken down by one of our chauffeurs, Sally," said Philip, "and two staff will have to go with her. Would you like to go? You probably should, in order to see what it's like and confer with the staff there about what she's able to do. I'd like to go too, if I can spare the time. We may have other clients who could go eventually."

For once everything went ahead without a problem, Rikki's parents had no objection, and as the day in April approached, I was looking forward to the trip almost as much as Rikki. I liked Philip's company. It would be nice to spend a whole day with him.

Rikki was so excited she could hardly sit still as her possessions were being loaded into the long station wagon by Denis, the chauffeur. At eight-thirty sharp, we were proceeding slowly down the driveway to the highway. Philip sat in front with the driver, Rikki and I in the back seat, the wheelchair, equipment and clothing occupied the space in the rear.

"Oh Sally," cried Rikki, groping for my hand. "I'm so glad to be getting out of this place, even if it's only for three weeks!"

"And leaving us?" I laughed.

"Well, not that. But you know what I mean."

"Yes, we know what you mean," said Philip, turning and smiling at me.

Rikki talked and sang the whole way down to Stemler, about a five hour drive. Stopping at a restaurant for lunch was a big treat and Rikki kept changing her mind about what she would have. I was less happy at the thought of the restaurant washroom, hoping that, being on a main highway, it would be accessible for wheelchairs. For this reason, we had made a point of stopping at a large service centre. But, to my dismay, the wheelchair would not even go through the washroom door.

Another customer, seeing our problem, said that there was a larger washroom in the Take-Out section. I wheeled Rikki over there, but it was locked. The only employee in sight was at the cash register. I asked her for the key to the Take-Out washroom. The woman was not prepared to help, and I was completely surprised at her response.

"That washroom is only open in the summer," she snapped. "She will just have to walk!"

I had to enlist Philip's help to carry Rikki in to the toilet. Denis had a back problem and was not allowed to lift residents.

There was a board on the wall with the names of the managers of the restaurant. I wrote down the particulars to lodge a complaint on behalf of others like Rikki.

We arrived at Palmer House in early afternoon. It had been a lovely day for Rikki. I described the building as we approached. It was new, with a modern circular design, large windows, attractive entrance and spacious, bright lobby. Denis left us for another errand while Rikki settled into her new home, and Philip and I enjoyed a cup of afternoon tea with some of the other residents. Rikki had soon made friends with Jane and Alec, both disabled with more severe cerebral palsy than Rikki. They told her about their recent engagement and wedding plans, and how arrangements had been made for them to share an apartment in the same residence, where they would both have the kind of care that they needed. Rikki was amazed that such disabled people could be allowed to be so normal.

She was delighted with her room, a single, with an accessible bathroom, to be shared with Jane next door. She was intrigued with the innovative plan of the building. The main corridor followed a circular design, an ideal arrangement for someone with severe visual handicap, and she felt immediately at home in the warm friendly environment.

The trip home gave us an opportunity we had never had to talk about things outside of work. I didn't know anything about Philip's private life, and I don't suppose he knew anything about mine. The people we worked with tended to be acquaintances, as opposed to friends, particularly if we lived in different towns. We were close to the same age, and both very interested in our professions.

I told Philip that I lived in the city, which meant an hour's drive each way every day, but I enjoyed the driving, because it gave me an uninterrupted time to plan my programs. Philip owned a house in town near the institution. He belonged to the local flying club nearby, and spent most of his spare time there.

"Why don't you move out here, Sally," he asked. "It must cost something to drive your car all this way every day."

"Yes," I replied. "But I belong to a riding club in the other direction, and spend most of my weekends there or at horse shows."

"So that's why you were able to start the riding program."

"Yes, but it was Dr. Ambrose who suggested it. I didn't know about the stable out here, and it hadn't occurred to me that we'd be able to have a program like this. We're so lucky to have an arena and a good instructor. Why don't you come out and see the program some day?"

"I'd like to. How about coming out to the flying club one day. I'll take you up for a spin."

"As long as it's not a tail-spin!"

It was about eleven o'clock when we arrived back at the institution, after stopping for dinner at a roadside restaurant. We thanked Denis for the trip and walked across the parking lot to our cars.

"Maybe our luck is changing, Sally. This is the break we were waiting for. I think Rikki will do well there".

"Rikki will make it now," I said. "Just you wait and see."

In May, while Rikki was still away, Dr. Piercey came again and was able to watch both the riding program and the gymnastics class that I had started in the gym. I knew that sooner or later someone was going to fall off a horse, especially when they started learning to trot over cavaletti, and I didn't want this to be a traumatic experience. To give them an idea of the height of the horse, I always insisted that all who were able should mount from the ground and for safety reasons, I would not allow any of them to be fastened in any way to the saddle.

The riders had one surprising characteristic in common, which must have been due to their blindness. They were all greatly stimulated by the experience, but none of them showed any fear. As a result, with reinforcement from the side-walkers, they trusted the instructor implicitly and followed her commands completely. Concepts like left and right, head up or down, open rein, forward position, heels down, were all new to them, but they learned them readily and were able to apply this to ward activities. None of them had any concept of the speed or pace of a horse, but then none of them had ever learned to run, jump, climb or use their muscles against resistance. Gradually strength, coordination and muscle tone improved, as well as morale.

I had been given permission to use the gym as long as I planned and directed the program myself, and enlisted the help of kinesiologists only if they were free. In spite of the reluctance of the physiotherapist to help, they actually wanted to help out, and many of them did.

The gym program consisted of an obstacle course, with mat work, somersaults, breakfalling, climbing the wall bars, climbing over the lowest level of the vaulting box, holding the handles of the vaulting horse while jumping on the springboard, then climbing over, and learning to run by trailing a hand along the wall. Flopping about on the trampoline was the greatest fun. It taught the gymnasts to move their bodies safely in space, and they loved it.

When I discovered that none of them knew how to pull against resistance I introduced weighted pulleys. They were all learning so rapidly that Mikaela suggested making a videotape of both the riding and the gym programs. She noticed the improvement in language skills too, and was impressed that Benny, our previously non-verbal resident, had started to talk in the program, and that Charlie was beginning to speak on his own, instead of remaining echolalic; always repeating only what someone else had said.

"I'm interested in your theory that there's a connection between gross motor activity and speech," Mikaela said as we walked back to the ward. "Your programs are all working well, and I'm impressed with the initiative and skill of the ward counselors. The results that you're getting show that you're offering the right programs. On the strength of their progress so far, how many would you say will outgrow the institution?"

I thought for a moment. "It's hard to say, Mikaela. We really didn't know when we started what response we would get. Chrissie has advanced the most, but Peer, in my opinion, has always been misplaced here and, of course, Rikki. And Peer and Rikki are very anxious to get out. The others don't really know what they're missing, or what's out there, because they've never lived anywhere else that they can remember. All the riders have made enormous gains. Even little Donny. He loves that pony that he rides each time, and it doesn't mind a bit when he hugs it with all his strength. We're beginning to wonder about Benny's real ability. He's much more aware now of what goes on in the ward than he's ever been… I think I could say that at least nine will outgrow the program this year. None of them are ready to manage outside yet, and it will be a long time before any of them could manage without some sort of support.

"There's something I'd like to ask you, Mikaela. Do you think, if we had chosen the residents for this ward at random, instead of going by the lists the counselors gave, we would be getting the same results?"

Mikaela thought for a moment. "That's something I've been wondering myself, Sally. There's a theory that meaningful activity is essential for development of the mind, and that mentally disabled people do better when they have a certain amount of physical activity. And that's why we have to start thinking about where these residents can go from here, and give the next lot a chance. We identified almost two hundred legally blind altogether, didn't we?

"Now there's something I want *you* to think about, Sally. Do you think you and Philip could get a committee together to study the possibilities of future placement for at least ten? Some could come from other institutions, not necessarily all from here. We'll have to create something, but then, you're accustomed to that, aren't you?"

I laughed. "Philip and I have been talking about this. Where should we start?"

"I've been thinking about it. They'll have to move out of the building. Maybe there's a smaller building on the grounds, or perhaps in town. Call me when you have some ideas and we can discuss it. And let me know when you want me to come again."

There was one member of staff on the blind ward who, in my opinion, showed exceptional insight into the problems of the blind residents and who seemed to know how to teach them better than the others. This was Betty Cameron, who had come to the ward with the final group of new residents. Betty had not worked with blind residents before in the institution, but it transpired that she had a blind brother. I was interested in Betty's approach to a problem, and I soon realized that her brother had given her an insight into the problems of blindness that the others did not have. Betty also had superior teaching skills and unlimited patience.

One day Betty asked permission to invite several residents to her home for tea. The first three to go were Chrissie, Peer and Harry. Roxanne, one of the new counselors, was helping to get them ready as I watched.

"Here Chrissie, put your coat on," Roxanne was saying. Betty walked over to Roxanne.

"I know you're in a hurry to get them ready, Roxanne, but may I make a suggestion?"

"Of course," said Roxanne, puzzled.

"You went to the cupboard, got Chrissie's coat for him, and asked him to put it on. Let's use this as an example of the difference between custodial care and rehab. Chrissie knows where the coat cupboard is and how to get there. Let's let him get his own coat from now on. And one other thing, Roxanne, you didn't tell Chrissie why he was putting his coat on, or where he was going. Preparation to go somewhere is as much a learning experience as going there, because it teaches anticipation, and that leads to planning, something these guys have never been able to do."

Roxanne looked at Betty for a few minutes, holding the coat. "I guess we're so used to doing it for them that we forget, Betty. You're right. But it's kind of hard when you know that they won't know what a private home is like until they get there."

"Yeah, think of it this way, Roxanne. Most of our residents have never had an opportunity to anticipate anything, or even to visualize something ahead of time. We have to teach them. And it doesn't matter at first whether what they anticipate is right or wrong, as long as they do it, because the next time they'll be able to anticipate more correctly. This is how they can learn to organize their behavior properly. Remember too, Roxanne, not to come up behind a blind person and touch him without any warning. This can produce a startle response, particularly if you grab him from behind. These are things we've all had to learn on this ward. Just look at the good results we're getting. It's really important for us to be consistent in what we teach. I hope you don't mind."

I thought to myself, "What a super staff we have here!"

The visits to Betty's house were the highlight of the week and each resident looked forward to being chosen to go. Several of them were surprised that Betty had her own bathroom and her own kitchen sink, but they wanted to know where the chapel and gymnasium were.

Each day we tried to plan some specific purposeful activity for them that was challenging without over-programming. Three headphones and an amplifier had been installed in the office, and residents were encouraged to listen to stories on cassettes whenever they felt like it. The tapes were made by volunteers and the stories were selected according to the comprehension and social maturity of the listener. I was pleased and surprised that Donny was becoming the best listener. Although he was fourteen years old, he particularly liked the story of "The Three Little Pigs", and listened to it over and over. At first he was just enjoying the sound of the reader's voice, but now he was beginning to understand the words and developing his own language from it.

I became aware of this one day when I overhead a visitor talking to Donny about his favourite story. She asked him what the little pig did when the wolf came down the chimney. Without hesitation Donny replied, "I guess he had roast wolf for breakfast."

I was elated. This was a real break-through for Donny. He was definitely developing his own language code. My only disappointment was that Mr. Nash, the Administrator, had never come to see our program.

Chapter 19

TEMPERED VICTORIES

"In journeys, as in life, it is a great deal easier to go downhill than up."
Charles Dickens

Rikki returned from Palmer House with enthusiastic accounts of her three weeks there. Most important of all, she was given a letter of recommendation that left no doubt about her ability to adjust to a community environment with appropriate support services.

Two ward counselors had been sent down to bring her back, so that they, too, could see this different environment and discuss Rikki's performance with the resource team when they got back.

Philip read the letter to the members of the team at our next meeting. It stated that Rikki was actually functioning above average among the thirty-two residents at the home, and that they would have no hesitation whatever in accepting her as a permanent resident if they did not have such a long waiting list from their own region. They recommended that, if it could be found, a smaller, more normal, community-based home would be more suitable for Rikki. There she would have more opportunity for independence than was offered at Palmer House, which is intended primarily for more severely disabled cerebral palsied residents who are less able to do much for themselves.

"May I suggest," said Philip, "that we send a copy of this letter to Rikki's parents and, with their permission, a copy to the director of Owen House in Windford, our nearest Cheshire Home, and request that she at least be put on their waiting list." This was unanimously approved. Then I suggested that Mikaela be invited to come again to discuss future plans for Special B.

As spring moved into summer, several things happened to disturb the daily routine of the institution, involving both me and Philip. Application had been made by Philip for Rikki's friend Lally to also have a three week trial period at Palmer House in Stemler, and in due course acceptance for Lally was received.

To Philip's dismay, he discovered that some of the counselors on Lally's ward had been persistently warning her against going, telling her that no one would know how to look after her there, and that she would be unhappy leaving everyone here. As Lally's fears mounted and the day of departure approached, Lally became mysteriously ill and had to be confined to bed.

Somehow word was leaked to Philip that Lally was being given medication to make her ill. Philip was so angry that he insisted that Lally depart on schedule, and that he go with her. All this was divulged to me upon Philip's return.

"Lally was beginning to recover when we got there," Philip was saying. "There is no question that she was being given medication to prevent her from leaving the institution."

"But Philip, the staff would have had to be pretty desperate to do a thing like that. Are you absolutely certain?"

"Absolutely, Sally. I'll lay my job on the line over this. Actually, it will probably put my job on the line. I don't expect any support."

"But if you're right, Philip, shouldn't you report it?"

"They would all cover it up, Sally. It's their jobs or mine, right? They see their jobs going out the window every time a good resident leaves. My job is becoming more and more impossible here every day."

"Mine too, Philip. I think the riding program is at an end. I really think that if Mr. Nash and the unit directors wanted to "scupper" the program, they would not go about it in any other way. The gym programs have been among the most successful ever offered, and yet we have had no end of obstacles and not one word of praise. Yesterday, I got a memo from Mr. Nash saying that no staff were to be spared for the riding program during the summer months when the high school students are not available. The summer is the very best time for the residents to enjoy the outdoors. And last week I was told that employees are no longer allowed to drive residents in their private cars."

"I hate to tell you this, Sally, but be prepared for another one. There's a new policy coming that says that residents are no longer allowed to go to private homes, except their own family home."

"Good heavens, Philip! Why? Does that mean that our blind residents can't go over to Betty Cameron's?"

"That's right. Apparently a parent complained because some years ago a female resident had been abused. Now all female residents are going to have to be signed out by women only, and accompanied by a female staff to their destination. They can't even be taken out by male members of their own families without a female going along."

"I don't believe it!" I exclaimed.

"It's all based on fear, Sally. That's the whole problem with this place… fear of job security, fear of incidents, fear of government power, and fear of peer power. They completely forget that we're dealing with people."

Mikaela came again, and helped the committee to draft a proposal for ten blind residents to move to a separate building on the grounds of the establishment, so that they could be trained in a more normal environment. The proposal was submitted, but in due course a memo arrived by way of response, stating that the proposed building was unsuitable for blind residents and would not pass fire standards. The proposal was therefore refused.

Almost the last straw for me was the removal of the trampoline, just as the residents were learning to move their bodies in space, a very necessary part of body image training. The reason given was that it was too dangerous, in spite of the fact that it was supervised by staff on all four sides and additionally padded.

It was just at that time, when I was ready to give up, that the good news arrived that Rikki had been accepted for a three month trial period at Owen House, the Cheshire Home in Windford. The selection committee had expressed some misgivings that Rikki might not fit in due to blindness, but also because she would be the only resident who had come from an institution, but they were willing to give her a chance.

That same day Mikaela telephoned. She had arranged for Philip and me to attend a meeting in Middleton, with representatives from other institutions, to discuss plans for a group home.

The first meeting was attended by representatives from all the institutions who were concerned about the problems with institutionalization for people with this type of disability, and consisted of two special education teachers, two social workers, one psychologist, one parent, an ophthalmologist, an optometrist, and the director of the national Agency for the Blind. I was the only occupational therapist.

After the meeting, I told Mikaela the good news about Rikki as well as the most recent set-backs in the gym program. "Never mind, Sally," she said, "That's good news about Rikki. So just carry on as best you can. We're off to a good start. At least three of the largest institutions are interested in our plans and want to be part of it, so we'll plan to have more meetings on a regular basis. Middleton is the most central location for everyone, so arrangements will be made for you and Philip if you would be willing to attend the meetings once a month."

"But what if Mr. Nash disagrees?"

"It will not be his decision, Sally. Tell your committee to consolidate their ideas. The next meeting will be in two weeks."

Although we all shared common concerns, agreement on specific issues was illusive. The meetings were long, arduous, and intensely involved with discussions about philosophy, basic goals, funding and location. There was agreement on the main objective, to find a better environment for the blind residents of our institutions, but no one seemed to have any clear idea of how this could be done. Not one person felt experienced enough to take the responsibility of leadership, so the chairperson had to change at each meeting. At first Philip and I were concerned that the meetings required an overnight trip for many of us without much being accomplished. The first three meetings were devoted mainly to selecting a suitable name for the home.

We were becoming aware that government funding for this sort of specialized project was bleak because of the apparent lack of encouragement from those in senior positions, and even suspicion on the part of the large established organizations serving people with developmental as well as visual disabilities. It was very much of a territorial thing. For this reason, it was important that our planning should be thorough, professional and realistic.

In the meantime, Philip proceeded with the arrangements for Rikki's move to Owen House, having received permission from her parents. This was not given without some reservation, for neither of Rikki's parents were in good health, their home was not wheelchair accessible, and they had never considered the possibility that she would ever live at home. They acknowledged that she was indeed their daughter, they loved her and were concerned for her future, but they were anxious about putting themselves in a position where she might become dependent on them, physically or financially, and they did not know how to express these fears.

Permission was granted for Rikki when it was carefully explained by Philip that, once removed from the institution, she would receive a disability pension. Rental costs at the home would be subsidized and paid by Rikki out of her disability pension, as well as food costs, leaving her a small amount for pocket money. It was also explained that I would be required to monitor her progress for the three month probationary period, and that any time within this period she could return to the institution.

Rikki was to move into Owen House the first of August. Philip had received reports that Lally had settled in well at Palmer House and that there was a possibility that she might be able to stay, because her family had been living for some time within that region.

For me, these victories were tempered by the thought that something would go wrong. A dream was about to be realized, and yet the smell of victory was not there. For the first time, I began to think about my own future.

Chapter 20

GATHERING CLOUDS

"The right to live is abused whenever it is not constantly challenged."
George Bernard Shaw

When one struggles against all odds towards a specific goal over a long period of time, one becomes so accustomed to the struggle, to not giving up, to holding tenaciously to a dream, that the sudden realization of that dream can come as a shock, and require a period of adjustment.

Rikki's acceptance at Owen House, albeit on trial, was the result of four years of training, planning, hoping and dreaming. It was a victory against defeatism, handicapism, and prejudice. And now there was no retreat, no turning back, the die was cast. Rikki knew without being told that this was her one big chance. It was a turning point in her life and she had to succeed. It was not a single handicap that had denied Rikki a normal life, but the result of a devastating combination of two handicaps that multiplied, like Helen Keller's, into a third and a fourth problem which disguised her true ability and prevented her from leading a normal life in a family home.

Rikki was also the victim of a social system that liked to classify people into tight little compartments, neatly labeled, with no room for anyone who did not fit. The blind belonged with the blind, the retarded with the retarded, the severely physically disabled with other physically disabled, and the elderly with the elderly. There was always the fear of duplication of services as well as total disregard for the problems of someone with multiple disabilities who might not fit any one label.

The terror and grief experienced by a totally blind person when placed on a ward with sighted, severely retarded people was beyond the comprehension of the people who made these decisions. And professionals who should have known better did not understand that lack of expressive ability did not indicate an equivalent absence of receptive language comprehension. Professionals were so pre-occupied with their own specialty that they seemed to have lost the ability to see or reason beyond it, or even to view their responsibility as having anything to do with problem solving on behalf of the whole patient.

Over a period of only four years Rikki had been assessed by more than thirty health professionals who were supposedly qualified. Nevertheless, there was no evidence that most of them had done anything to better her lot or alter her life in any way, and many had even attempted to impose further restrictions on her attempts at rehabilitation.

The day that Rikki was to move from the institution to Owen House I decided to take the day off and go, instead, to the group home to see how Rikki was settling in. When I arrived, I found Rikki's mother there ahead of me. Mrs. Chase, who was sorting Rikki's possessions on the bed, broke into a fit of crying when I arrived.

"Whatever is the matter?" I asked, alarmed. Rikki was sitting in her wheelchair beside the bed, her head down, silent.

"Just look what they've sent for Rikki to wear!" said her mother. "It's a disgrace! And we've been sending her good clothing for years."

I looked at the heaps of rumpled clothing taken from the over-stuffed paper grocery bags on the bed. Nothing had been pressed or folded, just stuffed into the shopping bags, but it was the type of clothing that appalled me. It was the middle of the summer heat wave, yet the clothing for Rikki to wear consisted of two heavy flannelette nightgowns, ten pair of discoloured underpants with stretched elastic, one tired-looking brassiere, four turtle-necked cotton pullovers that had once been white, two pair of red winter knee socks and two very short skirts that did not fit Rikki.

There was no light summer clothing, no light lingerie, no housecoat, no shorts or slacks, no dresses and no grooming equipment -- not even a toothbrush. Some clothing would have to be borrowed from the other residents until I or Mrs. Chase could outfit Rikki for the summer. I intended to lodge a strong complaint at the institution and promised to arrange to have Rikki's summer clothing sent as soon as possible. Her mother left in a state of anger and embarrassment. I spent an hour or so with the group home staff and promised to do something about the clothing situation immediately.

Sometimes, when working at the institution, I was reminded of Alice's Adventures In Wonderland. Nothing was ever what it seemed. What should have been logical was illogical. Procedures often seemed to be carried out backwards, and people who were used to the system seemed to have learned to respond in unpredictable ways.

I could spot all the Wonderland characters. I knew exactly who was the Doormouse, the March Hare, the Duchess, and even the Mad Hatter. I smiled as I turned my car once again up the long driveway. At least it was not dull, I thought. But why did I have such difficulty in predicting what was going to happen next? Perhaps it was just as well.

The ward seemed remarkably quiet as I entered. I noticed that Chrissie was sitting in his old position on the couch, rocking back and forth again.

"Chrissie's feeling sad to-day, Sally," said Ron. "You heard about the music lessons, didn't you?"

"No. What about them?"

"Canceled. Inter-departmental memo… came yesterday," said Ron. "Counselors are not allowed to teach music any more. The Rev's been relieved of his music staff."

"What do you mean, Ron?"

"I'll show you the memo Sally… here it is. Too bad. Chrissie was doing so well."

"So what's happened to Bob, he was teaching him and helping with the choir?"

"Put on kitchen duty… no choice… it's that or quit. No one's allowed to teach music any more. They're not paid for that."

"Well, hasn't anyone done anything about this?"

"What can we do? Stan says it's a new rule..."

I was dumbfounded. What was going to happen next? Rikki's clothing problems and now this. Mr. Nash had refused to see me on previous occasions because he insisted on speaking only to heads of departments, so I decided to write my own memo on both accounts immediately, and went up to my office. There would be copies to all unit directors, the administrator and also to Dr. Ambrose, although it was becoming clear to me that

Dr. Ambrose was becoming more and more in conflict with Mr. Nash, and had very little influence over anything affecting policy. I called Philip, but he was out, so I decided to have a talk with Dr. Ambrose anyway.

The doctor always had a calming effect on me. He was a slow moving man, and seemed resigned to the system. I wondered if I would ever be like that. I told him about Rikki's clothing problem and Chrissie's music lessons.

"Ah yes," he said, leaning back in his chair and re-packing his pipe. "It's very tiresome. Problems like these are always prevalent in institutions. It was hoped that the unit system would produce smaller hierarchies to avoid this sort of thing, but they were not organized properly. I would have liked to have seen a different system, but then, you see, we do what we can... or we move on to other things."

"Why do you stay, Doctor? How can you stand the system?"

"I ask myself the same question, sometimes, my dear. There are many here who have met that same brick wall head on. They stay 'til they can do no more, or until they have given up. And the others? You know what happens to them... too long on the tit, to use a vulgar expression. They're the ones you can't change any more. They've turned to stone. Sad. But don't let it discourage you. You've achieved a lot here, more than most. I hope you won't give up yet."

There was one question I had been wanting to ask Dr. Ambrose. It had some bearing on Rikki's management at Owen House. I knew that many of the female residents, including Rikki, were given regular injections of a contraceptive called Depo-Provera*, to prevent menstruation.[1]

"I read that it's been banned in the U.S., yet we're using it for many of our blind patients. Is it safe, Dr. Ambrose? I know Rikki has been getting it and I'm wondering if it's OK to continue."

"It was banned at one time for political reasons, not medical," said Dr. Ambrose. "We're convinced that it's perfectly safe or we would not be using it. It's the only answer for someone like Rikki, who wants to be more independent. Congratulations on finally getting her out. You've been doing excellent work. You'll keep me informed of her progress, and also about the ward, won't you?"

He did not say that he would try to help, but he was a good man. I felt sad for him, and wondered how long it would be before he gave up.

I sent the memos to the mail clerk and then walked over to Rikki's ward. I was prepared to offer to take her summer clothing in to Owen House if someone would pack it, but I was totally unprepared for the reaction to my complaints. Yvonne was on duty that day, sitting in the office.

"We particularly wanted Rikki to make a good impression, Yvonne," I said. "You've sent winter clothes, and it's the middle of summer. There's hardly anything she can wear. Who packed her clothing?"

---

[1] * "A recently published study in the United States, using data from New Zealand, Thailand, Kenya and Mexico, showed Depo-Provera does not increase the risk of breast cancer, a fear that led the U.S. Food and Drug Administration to ban the contraceptive from 1978 to 1992. Depo-Provera, which is manufactured by the American company Pharmacia & Upjohn Inc., is used by an estimated nine million women in 90 countries." Globe and Mail, Monday July 22, 1996

"Look around you, Sally. They're all still in winter clothing. The summer clothing was all ordered in May, and it hasn't arrived yet."

"Good Lord, what's happened to Rikki's last year's clothes, sent by her parents? ...Oh, don't bother answering, Yvonne, just tell me why there was only one bra, no slacks, no dress, no shorts, no tooth brush, no hairbrush..."

"You know about staffing on this ward, Sally," replied Yvonne, with a hint of whine in her voice. "Rikki's counselor is a male, and they're not so good at choosing female clothing. It was probably George. Doesn't know much about packing... Here he comes now, you can ask him yourself."

I had had dealings with George before. If I had to describe him in one word I would say tired, spelled L-A-Z-Y. George, predictably, saw nothing wrong with the clothing. "Rikki was told what was in them bags," he said, "and she approved everything herself."

I telephoned the results of my efforts to Rikki's mother and resolved to buy her some clothes myself if necessary. It had been another long day. Even Mikaela was not available. I decided to leave early. I had to get away.

Chapter 21

THE LAST STRAW

"Change is not made without inconvenience, even from worse to better."
Richard Hooker

During the next three months I made regular visits to Owen House as Rikki's liaison officer, and submitted the required progress reports. Rikki's determination to survive the probation period imposed an element of stress on everything that she did. She felt that her every move was being scrutinized and that the slightest mistake might result in being sent back.

She knew that she was different from the other residents. For the most part they, too, were wheelchair dependent due to injury or illness, but most of them were not congenitally disabled and had lived in normal home and school environments. They saw this as an interim placement, but Rikki longed for their acceptance. Her natural interest in people led her to make overtures of friendship and to show genuine concern for their problems. She lacked the social maturity to share many of their interests, because life in a normal community was so new to her, but she shared many of their concerns.

I had warned Rikki that transition to the community from the institution would not be easy. She insisted that she would face any alternative, no matter how difficult, but she had no idea what I meant. Her only goal was to escape to freedom -- freedom to make decisions about her own life, to make genuine, not paid friends, and to have her own money. She was unable to understand that this also meant the freedom to make mistakes, to endure physical discomfort, to accept responsibility, nor did she know what those responsibilities might be. Rikki did not yet understand that people who were paid to look after her were kind because that was their job, not because they had become personal friends.

One day, I asked her what had been her most important goal after leaving the institution. There was no hesitation. "Don't laugh, if I tell you," she said. "I've always wanted to have my own telephone, in my own room."

Many people had expressed concern about what Rikki would find to do in the home, how she would occupy her time. If I had any misgivings myself, I hid them in the back of my mind. No one at the institution seemed convinced that Rikki could have any role to play in the community. The only exception was the director of Owen House, who predicted no problem whatsoever.

The group home environment affected Rikki's behavior from the first day. The atmosphere was so different from an institution. The more relaxed routine, the normal conversation of the others, and their attitude towards her, combined to produce a kind of euphoria, and she was happier than she could ever remember. There were seven other residents at Owen House and usually only one or two counselors on duty. Residents helped with the household duties as much as they were able. They were all about Rikki's age chronologically, but not socially. Most went out to school or to work during the day and in the evening they would sit around the dining-room table and talk, watch television, or have their friends in.

By the end of the second month Rikki had a tutor from the local Board of Education, to continue with her French lessons, and she was looking forward to a recheck at Rehab. She had joined a church choir and had been enjoying visits to the shopping centre and the occasional concert. Her parents were able to make frequent visits.

But it was not always smooth sailing. Rikki's mother was going through an adjustment herself, and was only now able to regard her daughter as a thinking person. This sometimes resulted in arguments with the staff if she felt something was not clean enough, or if Rikki's hair had not been washed on a certain day, because she was still expecting her to have the same sort of custodial care she had in the institution.

The most serious problem occurred one day when the senior counselor telephoned me and suggested that possibly Rikki was not a suitable candidate for Owen House. She had thrown a tantrum in the evening and had kept the staff and some of the residents awake all night.

A volunteer had been taking her to church every Sunday, but last Sunday she waited all morning and the volunteer did not come. Eventually Rikki telephoned and spoke very rudely to her. The volunteer replied in the same tone, making it clear to Rikki that she would never take her again. I spoke to Rikki on the telephone. I explained to her that people are not always perfect, but also that she must not impose on volunteers or make demands on them beyond what they were prepared to do. I advised her to telephone and apologize to the woman for being rude to her. This is what set off the temper tantrum.

Rikki refused to call her, believing that the woman should apologize to her.

I then went over to Owen House for a short meeting with Rikki and the staff. I discussed with them the problems of transition that Rikki was going through. The staff was beginning to have second thoughts about the suitability of the home for her, and I wanted to dispel these fears if I could.

"She's had no experience with being assertive," I explained. "She's never been a normal teen-ager. She's never been allowed to have an argument with anyone."

I suggested that the staff might try not to take outbursts like this too seriously at first. Rikki needed to be allowed to sound off now and then without losing all her independence as a result. That was too great a punishment. But it was important to teach her the difference between appropriate and non-acceptable behavior. They agreed to give her another chance.

After the third month I was happy to report that Rikki had made a successful transition and had been accepted as a permanent resident at Owen House. My responsibility was therefore terminated and Rikki was officially discharged from the institution.

I took a two week holiday towards the middle of October. I felt the need for a break from the institution, partly to think seriously about my own future and to decide whether or not to make a change, and partly to renew my ability to make a useful contribution to the Special B team. I was aware that interest in the program was waning. With one or two exceptions, the staff were gradually loosing their original enthusiasm and beginning to show symptoms of that common malady called burn-out. In spite of the success of the programs, it was easy to fall back into the old ways, particularly when there was no specific goal in sight for the residents.

Philip and I continued to attend the meetings of the Planning Committee in Middleton once a month. The decision had been made to establish a home that would be central to the main institutions, but this ran into a snag when the District Working Group in Middleton refused our application because they were afraid that we would divert funding from their area. The committee advised me to try to obtain funding in the region where I lived, and to establish a Board of Directors there. I was appointed to approach the Cheshire Foundation regarding the possibility of membership and to seek their help in applying for government funding.

Subsequently, I met with some of the members of the Cheshire Foundation with Mikaela, and obtained the necessary papers to begin procedure for the acquisition of a government funded home for about ten residents. This was followed by meetings with the Assistant Deputy Minister and representatives from Cheshire to discuss eligibility for operational funding. I had learned before this meeting that, to date, Government funding for group homes had been restricted to either adults who were mentally retarded or people with severe physical disabilities, like quadriplegia. I knew that our clients did not fit the latter category, but I was very much against accepting the label of "retardation" or whatever the current term was. The Cheshire representatives agreed to support this.

I was impressed with their organization and discovered that there were over one hundred such homes throughout the world. They were originally established in England by World War II hero, Group Captain Leonard Cheshire, to provide affordable and accessible housing for war injured veterans. Although the movement had spread to Europe, Asia and Africa, as well as Canada, there was no record of one for blind disabled adult, and no one seemed to see any reason why there should not be such a home.

I returned to Maplegrove early in November, feeling elated about the meeting with the Cheshire committee and with Mikaela, and anxious to share the new information with Philip and the ward team. I had just arrived at my office when Claire called to ask me to report to her immediately.

"Have you been down to the ward B?" Claire asked. "Sit down for a moment. A few things have happened while you were away." I suddenly had a premonition that the news was not going to be good.

"First of all, Sally, Dr. Ambrose has resigned. He left without warning… just packed up and walked out."

"Oh, what a shame! I had a feeling that he would, though. I'm not really surprised. Sometimes I wondered why he hadn't left sooner. I think he was really a good doctor, but wasted here. Where did he go?"

"No one knows for sure, but someone said he had a good offer as a hospital manager."

"Good, I'm glad for him. What else happened?"

"One of the residents on your ward has eloped."

"Eloped? You mean he went out by himself? One of our blind residents? How would that be possible? Who was it?"

"He's O.K. It was a boy named Peer. Apparently he threw another tantrum on the ward earlier in the day, crashed a food wagon into the wall, narrowly missing one of the residents. One of the staff said that he was shouting, "I'm going to make you understand!" Later he conned a visitor into driving him into the city."

"But how would he know where to go? His parents don't live anywhere near here and Peer wouldn't know how to get around in the city."

"He went to the Agency for the Blind. They took him in and he says he's not coming back. I think he's actually within his rights to do that. I don't know what his family will think."

"Well, isn't that something! Good for Peer! He always wanted to get out. Maybe he'll be OK. But things go in threes, Claire. I hope nothing else happened."

"I'm saving the worst for the last, Sally," said Claire. "You're not going to like this. It all happened overnight last week with no warning. The staff is seething mad, and they're probably going to blame you, so be prepared."

"Blame me? What for? Can't I even go away on a holiday? What's happened Claire?"

"You know E Ward, across the hall from Special B? Well, it's now a new blind ward."

"You mean they moved Special B?"

"No. They collected twenty-five or thirty blind residents from the other wards and moved them all on Sunday into E and moved the E residents to other wards. The same E staff are still there, totally untrained to work with the blind, and they don't even know the names of the residents -- no IDs, no extra clothing -- it's an absolute shambles!"

"But Claire, how can they do that? Didn't they learn anything from what we were doing on B?"

"That's the next thing, Sally. The Special B staff is supposed to be teaching E ward, so they're all going out of their minds too."

"I don't believe this Claire. How could they do a thing like this? They've put E staff in an impossible position and it will ruin Special B. Damn it, Claire! I'm fed up with this place! Every time you think you've succeeded at building something good it's knocked down."

"You'll have to go down and help them, Sally. Some of the staff have quit. I don't know what you can do. Come and see me at lunch time."

I knew who was probably behind this latest development. There were a number of people with a certain amount of power in the institution who were able to make sudden decisions like this and yet remain anonymous. This subversive element was like a kind of "Mafia" that inspired fear in anyone who attempted to question authority. As I walked briskly, yet reluctantly, towards the unit I reflected on the many obstacles I had encountered since coming to this institution. Casual visitors would get a completely false impression of what it was really like. It would even be difficult to explain to them why the work was so stressful.

It was not the fault of any one person in particular, it was the entire system that was wrong because it allowed such things to happen. It was almost what might have been described as an exponential situation, where any one element was not dangerous in itself, but collectively they produced a disaster.

The situation that awaited me on ward E was most certainly a disaster. The noise, the seething movement of people, the expressions of anger and despair on the faces of the staff, the odor, all combined to produce panic and hopelessness.

"You'd better not come in here Sally, if you know what's good for you. Did you plan all this and then walk out and dump it on us? If you did, you're never going to forget it!" Jim Cowan had always been a quiet, mild-mannered man, but today he had changed.

"Jim, I knew nothing whatever about this until twenty minutes ago. I just can't believe what has happened."

"Right. Well, we'd better let the staff know that, because they're plenty mad. How does anyone think we can look after this lot. We don't know any of them. Their records haven't even come yet, we don't know what medication they're on, and they've been here since Sunday night."

"Do you mean to tell me that they were all moved on the week-end, with week-end staff on duty?"

"That's right. Don is supposed to be ward sup. here and he wasn't even told. All our residents were moved onto the other wards and these blind guys moved in, in their place. If you're not behind this Sally, who the Hell is? Don has already quit… just walked out… and we don't blame him."

No one had any time to talk. One man was running around the ward naked, a counselor trying to persuade him to stop to put his clothes on. Another was urinating against the wall. Several were still in bed, some huddled on the floor in the corner of the room. There were unmade beds, articles of clothing on the floor, basins of water and towels and a continual buzzing of sound as everyone moved about in the huge open crowded room.

I left the ward and walked across the hall to Special B. Howard was in his office.

"For God's sake, Howard, what happened? Who's responsible for this fiasco?"

"They're all blaming you at this point Sally. But wait. Don't get upset. I know it wasn't you. I think I know what happened, but no one is telling. Stanley has been having a few problems with some of the others. Don't quote me, but Stanley's under the gun. I can't say anything more. You know how it is. But you know what it's going to do to us. For one thing, it's depleted my staff already, just as we were getting somewhere with the program. I don't know what I can do Sally. Do you think Dr. Piercey could help?"

I called Mikaela from Howard's office, but she was out of town for the week. Howard produced a pot of coffee and I told him of the plans for a Cheshire Home.

"Maybe some of your staff could be employed at the home, Howard. At least, if we got it, it would give them something to work towards."

"Yeah, and how many years will that take, Sally? You're still wearing rose-coloured glasses."

"Yes Howard, I guess I am." I left the ward and went upstairs. I had to find Philip.

Chapter 22
ENDINGS AND BEGINNINGS

"And not by eastern windows only, when daylight comes, comes in the light, in front the sun climbs slow, how slowly, but westward look, the land is bright."
Say Not the Struggle Not Availeth,
Arthur Hugh Clough

I handed in my resignation at Maplegrove the following Monday, to become effective in the required two weeks time. I knew this was the expected and hoped-for response, and I was finally convinced that to stay any longer would not produce any positive results. The "coup" on ward E was the final stroke of defeat. Yet it was not really a defeat.

"You've just gone as far as you can here," Philip said. "We all know that any institution has limits. You are the type of person who needs to see results for job satisfaction. Most people here have no hope of working that way. They put in their day and get their pay cheque. You've reached the point where you have to totally change the environment for these guys, and you've finally realized that you can't do it if you stay here. So go for it."

"I don't know Philip. I would never have been able to go this far without you and Mikaela and some of the staff. What about you? Are you going to leave too?"

"Not for a while. I still have a few things to do. But you go ahead. Maybe I'll join you later. We're both still on the Middleton Planning Committee. I'll see you there -- if they don't prevent me from going."

"Philip, it would be so easy to give up, wouldn't it? But how can I let all those guys down, when they've done so well? And if I don't keep trying, all the work we've done in the past three years will be wasted, and they'll all revert back to where they were when this program started."

"I agree with you, Sally, and I'll help all I can, but you're the key person now. You'll have to work from a community base, not from here. I think what we need is a home with a more normal environment and a staff who are able to teach life skills."

"But Philip, I don't know how I can do that and hold down a job too. And the cost of traveling back and forth to Middleton will be expensive when I can't be on an expense account... I've been thinking though, and it's only just a theory, but when these residents became purposefully occupied, they began to learn, and their communication skills improved. Before, they were occupying themselves with deviant behavior, or behavior that was not socially normal. Do you think that if we had chosen them at random for the special program, instead of taking the staff recommendations, we would have had the same results? Am I right in thinking that when the program ceases to be meaningful they'll all revert back to where they were? What would it have been like for you or me, at their age, to have been blind and placed in an environment like this?"

Philip was silent for a minute. "I've wondered the same thing, Sally. What would you think of starting the first home near where you live? Maybe there could be another one in Middleton. We have enough residents here for the first home."

"Yes, that sounds possible, but the funding agencies are all in Middleton as well as the government offices and the Cheshire organization."

"Yes, but there's also more competition for funds there. It's a big city. You might actually stand a better chance in a smaller city like Windford, where there's less demand for this type of funding."

"Philip, you're talking absolute nonsense. I can't do this. I don't know anything about starting a home. And it would take an enormous amount of time. How could I afford to do it?"

"You couldn't just let it drop, Sally. We did get Rikki out, and Peer has "sprung" himself. They'll never come back. But what about the others?"

"Two, Philip? Out of how many?"

"We can't save the world, I know. But if we could only make an example with this one home, maybe the government would follow up with more. And there's another reason why the government might support it. It would cost less. When you think of the staff in this place; the maintenance people, the office staff, the cooks and kitchen staff, the cleaners, not to mention all the senior staff who don't even have contact with the residents, and on top of that, the cost of heating alone... It's bound to cost much more here than group homes. So don't give up. Mikaela will persuade the ministry to back you."

"Yes, but there's an election coming up. What if the whole government changes and Mikaela's out of a job?"

"She won't be, even if it does change. Come on Sally. You're just thinking of obstacles. Come to one more meeting in Middleton, make a proposal, and I'll support you."

* * *

The staff had a party for me on my last day, complete with a party table cloth, fancy cakes, tea and coffee. Everyone was so nice that I began to feel sad about leaving and wondered if I was doing the right thing. Had I expected too much? Everyone signed a card, wishing me the best for the future, and Claire presented me with a gift wrapped in pretty paper and ribbon. I opened it to find a photograph album, amid applause from the on-lookers.

Just then a knock was heard at the door and someone brought a note addressed to me. I excused myself and opened the letter, thinking it might be something important. There was a small card attached to a letter of recommendation. The card read, "Just thought you might have some use for this. Good luck." It was signed "Peter Ambrose." I felt a lump in my throat as I tucked the letter into my pocket.

The sun was low in the sky and dancing on the windshield as I drove down the long driveway for the last time. The blind residents had not really understood why I was leaving. They were so accustomed to having people leave that they might not have felt that this was unusual. Would they think that I had given up like so many other innovative programs that had been started and never finished at the institution? Or was what appeared to be a lack of concern really a reflection of lack of control over events, a certain helplessness that comes of knowing that what one says or does will make no difference.

My thoughts went back to my first day at Maplegrove, and to how much my expectations had changed since that day. I wondered if I would have stayed so long if I had known ahead what to expect. Probably not. Yet I would not have missed this experience for anything in the world.

I thought of the wonderful people I had met during this time, of Dr. Piercey… Mikaela, my advisor and mentor throughout, who had such insight into the problems of these young people, and who always gave such good advice, and Dr Ambrose, Rikki, Peer, Chrissie, Harry… such likable, kind, forgiving young people. And I thought of Philip, and how I would miss him, and not in the least, of the eager, hard-working resourceful ward staff, I would miss them too.

But all that was behind me now. It was like starting a new chapter in my life. I knew then that I was not going to give up. I would have to find a way.

Postscript

"Thanks to the help from a concerned community, there are now over 24 Cheshire homes in Ontario, providing accommodation for people with disabilities, but thousands are on the waiting list. The annual cost to the taxpayer for an individual in a chronic care institution is at least $146,000. In a Cheshire facility it is less than $60,000, and makes the lives of people with physical disabilities productive and promising."

The Cheshire Homes Foundation
Toronto, Canada,
April, 1995

Epilogue

It is now over thirty years since "Rikki" escaped from the institution. A true pioneer, she helped create many of the services that are now available for people like her.

Rikki subsequently spent ten years in a group home in the community before she was accepted for an independent living co-operative apartment with support services. During that time, she completed her grade nine French course with honours and attended three high schools with a modified curriculum, including English, music and life skills.

Always having a goal ahead of her, Rikki's first objective - to have a telephone in her room - soon expanded to a high-tech telephone, stereo, and security system that she describes in engineering terminology. Her attractive, spacious apartment is designed for wheelchair users according to the latest Government specifications. She uses a hydraulic bath lift and has support staff that prepares her meals, does the laundry and helps with light housekeeping and clothes selection. Otherwise, Rikki is essentially independent, manages her own affairs, buys her own groceries, regularly attends theatre, church, concerts and travels about by Para Transpo.

Her specially designed apartment has allowed her to live alone and to be more independent than the small group home, (Owen House) that was not designed for independent wheelchair mobility. As a result, she has been able to benefit from occupational therapy training in life skills, and is much less dependent on staff assistance than ever before.

Rikki receives a disability pension that allows her to manage her own affairs, do her own banking and pay her rent and living expenses. The cost to the government is less than half the cost of keeping her in an institution. She seldom spends a day at home, travels to other cities occasionally, and was a guest speaker for an organization in Newfoundland. She belongs to several clubs, has a half-time volunteer job as a telephone receptionist and has many friends and a cat. A few years ago she attended a conference in London, England, as a Cheshire Homes representative, and was introduced to the Queen. Rikki has a keen interest in music. She is now in her fourth year of music appreciation at a local university, and has a large collection of cassette tapes and C.D.s. She obtains 'Talking Books' on cassette through the local public library where a volunteer helps her with book selection.

"Peer" discharged himself too soon, before there were suitable community services available for him. He learned Braille at the institution, but unfortunately had not been taught any behavioural or marketable skills that would help him in a hostile world. As a result, his adjustment was difficult. He never returned to the institution.

Two years after Rikki's move to the community, and too late for Peer, funding was obtained to open the first Cheshire Home in North America for blind adults with additional disabilities. Renovating and operating costs, such as staff salaries and the mortgage, were supplied by the Government Services Department for disabled citizens. Furnishings were supplied by donations from the community. The first ten residents came from two of the largest institutions, most of them from our special ward. The business management of the home is under the direction of a qualified and capable volunteer Board of Directors.

Alterations to the home, to accommodate ten residents, were designed to eliminate hazards and promote maximum independence, but have remained as close as possible to a normal family home. Staff was selected according to teaching ability and motivation to encourage independence. After an assessment period, mainly to assure that the applicant would not be a danger to self or others in the home, and would be likely to benefit by living there, all were assured that this would be their home for as long as they wished to stay.

This home, and a second that followed five years later, have been an unqualified success. Psychological testing by the government over the first two years showed statistically significant improvement in general knowledge, behavioural, and life skills among all ten residents. Although all residents will not become as independent as Rikki, all are actively involved in community activities, school or training programs and some are now employed in the community. They all help out in the home as they are able.

"Chris", who had been institutionalized from the age of ten and moved into the group home at age nineteen, won a scholarship during his last special education year at a city high school. In addition to being a competent musician and playing several instruments, he now has a full time job with union wages. Another resident showed marked improvement in communication skills when it was discovered that he had a double hearing loss that was corrected by hearing aids. Speech therapy has helped another to speak more clearly, so that he can now be understood. A third resident's behaviour improved dramatically following intensive medical treatment that eliminated most of the medication she had been on over a period of several months. Another resident has learned to play the organ well enough to play, occasionally, for services at a local church.

Five to seven years were required for most of those first residents to complete the process of de-institutionalization and learn normal living skills, such as appropriate speech and language, good manners, acceptable dress, and basic marketable work skills. Chris, like Rikki, now lives in his own apartment but he, like all the others who may eventually move into a more independent situation, will always be able to look upon this as their family home. The friends he made at the home will always remain his cherished friends, and the staff will always be a resource for him when needed.

It is important for funding organizations to understand the reasons why this type of group home, with built-in teaching programs that expand into community resources, has succeeded as an alternative to institutionalization. Nevertheless, they should be careful not to fall into the trap of over-protectionism, isolation from the community and the hiring of staff who lack the necessary skills and patience. There is always a danger that a group home could become another institution.

It is unnatural for humans to be physically and mentally idle. Enforced idleness in both humans and animals can lead to deviant behaviour. When total blindness is a factor, adjustment to blindness in a sighted world has to be taught. Starting in infancy, a blind baby must be taught to use his other senses of hearing, balance, touch, taste and smell to compensate for the loss of vision.

This instruction is even more important if the person has an additional disability. Even if he has a learning problem, or is wheelchair dependent, his training and education must include orientation to his surroundings along with independence in mobility. Furthermore, where possible, he should learn adequate reading and mathematics skills with appropriate technology, effective use of language, and good social skills.

Intelligence testing that does not take into consideration the factor of blindness, particularly along with impaired speech and language comprehension and social awareness, is invalid and misleading. Meaningful normal activity, exercise, problem solving, a continual learning environment, a sense of belonging and a sense of worth that concentrates on an individual's ability rather than disability, can produce miraculous results. This is what Helen Keller meant when she said "There is no handicap in blindness, the handicap is in idleness", and the improvement in the quality of life is immeasurable.

CPSIA information can be obtained at www.ICGtesting.com
Printed in the USA
LVOW081844170112

264291LV00001B/96/P

9 781602 641693